Clinic Handbook of Gastroenterology

Clinic Handbook of Gastroenterology

John L. H. Wong
Research Fellow, Endoscopy Unit
Royal Cornwall Hospital, Truro, Cornwall

Iain Murray
Consultant Physician/Gastroenterologist
Royal Cornwall Hospital, Truro, Cornwall

S. Hyder Hussaini
Consultant Physician/Gastroenterologist
Royal Cornwall Hospital, Truro, Cornwall

Harry R. Dalton
Consultant Physician/Gastroenterologist
Royal Cornwall Hospital, Truro, Cornwall

A CIP catalogue record for this book is available from the British Library.

ISBN 1 85996 053 7

BIOS Scientific Publishers Ltd
9 Newtec Place, Magdalen Road, Oxford OX4 1RE, UK.
Tel. +44 (0)1865 726286. Fax. +44 (0)1865 246823
World Wide Web home page: http://www.bios.co.uk/

Distributed exclusively in the United States, its dependent territories, Canada, Mexico, Central and South America, and the Caribbean by Springer-Verlag New York Inc, 175 Fifth Avenue, New York, USA, by arrangement with BIOS Scientific Publishers Ltd, 9 Newtec Place, Magdalen Road, Oxford OX4 1RE, UK.

Important Note from the Publisher
The information contained within this book was obtained by BIOS Scientific Publishers Ltd from sources believed by us to be reliable. However, while every effort has been made to ensure its accuracy, no responsibility for loss or injury whatsoever occasioned to any person acting or refraining from action as a result of information contained herein can be accepted by the authors or publishers.

The reader should remember that medicine is a constantly evolving science and while the authors and publishers have ensured that all dosages, applications and practices are based on current indications, there may be specific practices which differ between communities. You should always follow the guidelines laid down by the manufacturers of specific products and the relevant authorities in the country in which you are practising.

Production Editor: Andrew Watts.
Typeset by Saxon Graphics Ltd, Derby, UK.
Printed by TJ International Ltd, Padstow, UK.

Contents

1 Dyspepsia

John Wong

2 Dysphagia

Diana Stone

3 Jaundice

Jon Mitchell

4 Iron Deficiency Anemia

Hyder Hussaini

5 Rectal Bleeding

Christine Bloor

6 Abdominal Pain

Sunil Samuel

7 Abnormal Liver Function Tests

Hyder Hussaini

8 Change in Bowel Habit: Constipation/Unexplained Diarrhea

Joy Worthington and John Wong

9 Weight Loss/Nausea and Vomiting

Iain Murray

10 Screening

Sunil Samuel and John Wong

11 Inflammatory Bowel Disease

John Wong

12 Irritable Bowel Syndrome

John Wong

13 Chronic Viral Hepatitis

Hyder Hussaini

14 Nonviral Chronic Liver Disease

Hyder Hussaini

15 Celiac Disease

Iain Murray

16 Nutrition

Mark McAlindon

17 Developing a Successful Gastrointestinal Service

Harry Dalton, Hyder Hussaini and Iain Murray

18 Patient Information

Harvey Dymond

19 Teaching in Gastroenterology

Harry Dalton, David Levine and Hyder Hussaini

20 Quality Assurance in Gastroenterology

Iain Murray

21 Radiology and the Gastroenterology Team

Richard Farrow and Giles Maskell

22 Palliation of Gastrointestinal Symptoms

Simon Noble

Abbreviations

5-ASA	5-aminosalicylic acid
5HT	serotonin
6-MP	6-mercaptopurine
AFP	alpha-fetoprotein
AGA	American Gastroenterological Association
AIDS	acquired immunodeficiency syndrome
ALD	alcohol-related liver disease
ALP	alkaline phosphatase
ALT	alanine transaminase (alanine aminotransferase)
AMA	antimitochondrial antibody
ANA	antinuclear antibodies
ANCA	anticytoplasmic antibodies
anti-dsDNA	antibody directed against double-stranded DNA
anti-HBc	antibody to HBcAg
anti-HBe	antibody to HBeAg
anti-HBs	hepatitis B surface antibody
anti-ssDNA	antibody directed against single-stranded DNA
APC	adenomatous polyposis coli
ASCA	anti-*Saccharomyces cerevisiae* antibody
AST	aspartate transaminase (aspartate aminotransferase)
bDNA	branched DNA
BMD	bone mineral density
BMI	body mass index
BSG	British Society of Gastroenterology
CBT	cognitive behavioral therapy
CCK	cholecystokinin
CD	Crohn's disease
CHI	Commission for Health Improvement
COX-2	cyclo-oxygenase 2
CRP	C-reactive protein
CRS	catheter-related septicemia
CT	computed tomography
CTC	computed tomography cholangiography
cusum	cumulative sum
DDF	Digestive Disorders Foundation
DEXA	dual emission X-ray densitometry
EATCL	enteropathy-associated T-cell lymphoma
EBV	Epstein–Barr virus
ECG	electrocardiogram
EGD	esophagogastroduodenoscopy
ELISA	enzyme-linked immunosorbent assay

EMAB/EMA	endomysial antibodies
ERC	endoscopic retrograde cholangiogram
ERCP	endoscopic retrograde cholangiopancreatography
ESR	erythrocyte sedimentation rate
EUS	endoscopic ultrasound
FAP	familial adenomatous polyposis
FBC	full blood count
FD	functional dyspepsia
GERD	gastroesophageal reflux disease
GGT	gamma-glutamyltransferase
GH	genetic hemochromatosis
GI	gastrointestinal
GMC	General Medical Council
GP	general practitioner
H_2 antagonist	histamine receptor antagonist
HACA	human antichimeric antibody
HAV	hepatitis A virus
HBcAg	hepatitis B core antigen
HBeAb	hepatitis B e antibody
HBeAg	hepatitis B e antigen
HBsAg	hepatitis B surface antigen
HBV	hepatitis B virus
HCC	hepatocellular carcinoma
HCV	hepatitis C virus
HDV	hepatitis delta virus
HEV	hepatitis E virus
HIAA	5-hydroxy-indoleacetic acid
HIV	human immunodeficiency virus
HMPAO	hexamethyl propylenamine oxine
HNPCC	hereditary nonpolyposis colon cancer
HP	*Helicobacter pylori*
HPN	home parenteral nutrition
HRT	hormone replacement therapy
IBD	inflammatory bowel disease
IBS	irritable bowel syndrome
IDA	iron deficiency anemia
IFNa	interferon alpha
Ig	immunoglobulin
INR	international normalised ratio
IVU	intravenous urogram
JAG	Joint Advisory Group on Gastrointestinal Endoscopy
JVP	jugular venous pressure
LFT	liver function test
LKM	liver kidney microsomal antibody

LES	lower esophageal sphincter
MRCP	magnetic resonance cholangiopancreatography
MRI	magnetic resonance imaging
MSI	microsatellite instability
NACC	National Association for Colitis and Crohn's Disease
NAFLD	nonalcoholic fatty liver disease
NASH	nonalcoholic steatohepatitis
NCEPOD	National Confidential Enquiry into Peri-operative Deaths
NICE	National Institute for Clinical Excellence
NSAIDs	nonsteroidal anti-inflammatory drugs
p-ANCA	perinuclear antineutrophil cytoplasmic antibody
PBC	primary biliary cirrhosis
PCR	polymerase chain reaction
PEG	percutaneous endoscopic gastrostomy
Peg	polyethylene glycol
PPI	proton pump inhibitor
PSC	primary sclerosing cholangitis
PTC	percutaneous transhepatic cholangiography
PTH	parathyroid hormone
RIBA	recombinant immunoblot assay
SLA	soluble liver antigens
SLE	systemic lupus erythematosus
SMA	smooth muscle antibody
SO	sphincter of Oddi
SSRI	selective serotonin reuptake inhibitors
TNFα	tumor necrosis factor α
TPMT	thiopurine methyltransferase
tTG	tissue transglutaminase
U&Es	urea and electrolytes
UC	ulcerative colitis
UDCA	ursodeoxycholic acid
VMA	vanillylmondelic acid

Contributors

Christine Bloor BSc(Hons), PGCE, ACMI
Clinical Specialist Radiographer,
Royal Cornwall Hospital, Truro, Cornwall
TR1 3LJ

Harry Dalton BSc, D.Phil, FRCP,
Dip Med Ed
Consultant Physician/Gastroenterologist,
Royal Cornwall Hospital, Truro, Cornwall
TR1 3LJ

Harvey Dymond BSc, RGN
Research Nurse, Endoscopy Unit,
Royal Cornwall Hospital, Truro, Cornwall
TR1 3LJ

Richard Farrow BSc, MRCP, FRCR, PGCE
Consultant Radiologist,
Royal Cornwall Hospital, Truro, Cornwall
TR1 3LJ

S. Hyder Hussaini DM, FRCP, PGCE
Consultant Physician/Gastroenterologist,
Royal Cornwall Hospital, Truro, Cornwall
TR1 3LJ

David Levine DM, FRCP, PGCE
Consultant Physician/Gastroenterologist,
West Cornwall Hospital, Penzance,
Cornwall TR18 2PF

Mark McAlindon B Med Sci, DM, FRCP
Consultant Gastroenterologist,
Royal Hallamshire Hospital, Glossop
Road, Sheffield S10 2JF

Giles Maskell MRCP, FRCR
Consultant Radiologist,
Royal Cornwall Hospital, Truro, Cornwall
TR1 3LJ

Jonathan Mitchell BM, MRCP
Clinical Fellow, Institute of Liver Studies,
Kings College Hospital, Bessemer Road,
London SE5 9RS

Iain Murray BSc(Hons), DM, MRCP
Consultant Physician/Gastroenterologist,
Royal Cornwall Hospital, Truro, Cornwall
TR1 3LJ

Simon Noble MRCP, Dip Pall Med
Specialist Registrar in Palliative Medicine,
Holmetower Marie Curie Centre,
Bridgeman Road, Vale of Glamorgan
CR64 3YR

Sunil Samuel MBBS, MRCP
Specialist Registrar in Gastroenterology,
Royal Cornwall Hospital, Truro, Cornwall
TR1 3LJ

Diana Stone B Med Sci, MBBS, MRCP
Research Registrar, Gastrointestinal Unit,
Royal Cornwall Hospital, Truro, Cornwall
TR1 3LJ

John L. H. Wong MBBCh, MRCP
Research Fellow, Gastrointestinal Unit,
Royal Cornwall Hospital, Truro, Cornwall
TR1 3LJ

Joy Worthington MBBCh, MRCP
Specialist Registrar in Gastroenterology,
North Devon District Hospital,
Barnstaple, Devon EX31 4JB

Preface

This book offers a practical guide in the gastroenterology outpatient clinics. The focus is on the approach to investigations for patients presenting with common gastrointestinal symptoms. This is supplemented by essential up to date clinical information which will be helpful in specialised clinics, and is aimed to meet the needs of Senior House Officers and Specialist Registrars. The sections on management, quality issues and education should be particularly useful for senior Specialist Registrars and newly qualified consultants. We hope non-specialist doctors will also find the handbook useful.

We are grateful to Mrs Jenny Harris for her help in typing the manuscript. We wish to thank Dr Helen Fellows who took the photograph of St Ives (Figure 17.1), Dr Robin Teague for his comments on Chapter 19 and Dr Sue Turner for agreeing to the use of her cusum chart (Figure 19.1).

We also wish to thank our publishers BIOS, particularly Dr Katie Deaton and Andrew Watts, for their help and support.

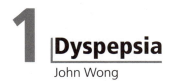

1 Dyspepsia

John Wong

Introduction

Dyspepsia has been defined as abdominal pain or discomfort centered in the upper abdomen or epigastrium. The term is not a diagnosis in its own right. It has been used to refer to various symptoms including upper abdominal fullness, retrosternal pain, early satiety, bloating, anorexia, nausea or vomiting. Patients with typical or predominant positional dependent heartburn have symptomatic gastroesophageal reflux disease (GERD) until proven otherwise and should not be labeled as dyspeptic.

Epidemiology

Dyspepsia is a common problem in the general population, with an estimated prevalence of 23–41% (GERD included) in most industrialized countries. Only about a quarter of those who experience dyspeptic symptoms seek medical attention. This accounts for about 4% of all family practice consultations in the UK. The reason for consultation is probably related to the symptom severity or frequency, fear of malignant diagnosis, underlying anxiety or other psychosocial factors. Investigations for dyspepsia usually result in diagnosis of GERD in about 20–40% of patients. Around 10–20% have endoscopic evidence of reflux esophagitis, while 15–20% may have peptic ulcer disease (gastric or duodenal ulcers), including duodenitis. Dyspepsia symptoms are frequently attributed to gastritis although these correlate poorly with histological findings of gastritis. Less than 1% have a diagnosis of gastric malignancy. Other causes of organic dyspepsia include pancreatic and biliary disorders, intolerance to medications, parasitic infection and systemic disorders such as diabetes mellitus, which can be associated with nausea and upper gastric dysmotility.

Management approach for patients without previous investigations

Only 10% of patients in the UK attending their general practitioner (GP) with dyspepsia will be referred for hospital consultation or investigations.

Alarm features

These include unintentional weight loss, iron deficiency anemia, gastrointestinal (GI) bleeding, dysphagia, odynophagia, previous gastric surgery, previous gastric ulcer, therapy with nonsteroidal anti-inflammatory drugs (NSAIDs), persistent vomiting, epigastric mass, suspicious findings from barium meal investigation, or epigastric pain severe enough to cause hospitalization. Early or urgent endoscopy is indicated.

Early endoscopy

Proponents of early endoscopy for all patients with dyspepsia argue that early endoscopy enables accurate diagnosis and detection or exclusion of gastric malignancy. However, the prevalence of gastric cancer is low and declining worldwide, with an incidence of less than 10 per 100 000 population in most western industrialized countries. One randomized study compared immediate investigation (prompt endoscopy) with empirical therapy (histamine 2 receptor antagonist) for patients with dyspepsia. Of the patients randomized to empirical therapy, 66% required endoscopy anyway in the first year of follow-up. Decreased drug cost and increased patient satisfaction was observed in the early endoscopy group. Cost analysis favored early endoscopy over empirical medical treatment when all medical and social costs were considered.

Test-and-treat strategy (see Figure 1.1)

New onset of symptoms at the age of 45 and above, and the use of NSAIDs, increases the likelihood of finding endoscopic abnormalities. The British Society of Gastroenterology (BSG) and the American Gastroenterological Association (AGA) include these as indications for endoscopy in dyspeptic patients.

Noninvasive testing for *Helicobacter pylori* (HP) has been recommended as an approach to increase diagnostic yield and rationalize the use of endoscopy. Lack of HP infection is a good predictor for the absence of peptic ulcer disease or gastric cancer. Conversely, 20–50% of dyspeptic patients who test positive for HP will have evidence of underlying ulcer disease or duodenitis. This approach is dependent on easily accessible and accurate HP tests, especially for primary care physicians. It has not been shown to decrease endoscopy workload in prospective clinical studies.

More recently, a 'test and treat' strategy has been suggested. Patients who test positive for HP are given a course of HP eradication therapy if there are no alarm symptoms or new onset of symptoms at age 45 and above. Endoscopy is restricted for failure of symptomatic response or relapse of dyspeptic symptoms after eradication therapy. The rationale is that effective HP eradication will treat peptic ulcer disease and may benefit patients with functional dyspepsia (FD), without the need for further investigations.

HP infection can be diagnosed noninvasively by serology, or by ^{14}C or ^{13}C urea breath test. Patients are normally advised to discontinue proton pump inhibitors (PPIs) for at least 2 weeks prior to the breath test. A typical triple therapy HP eradication scheme consists of two antibiotics (clarithromycin 500 mg, metronidazole 400 mg/tinidazole 500 mg or amoxicillin 1 g) and one

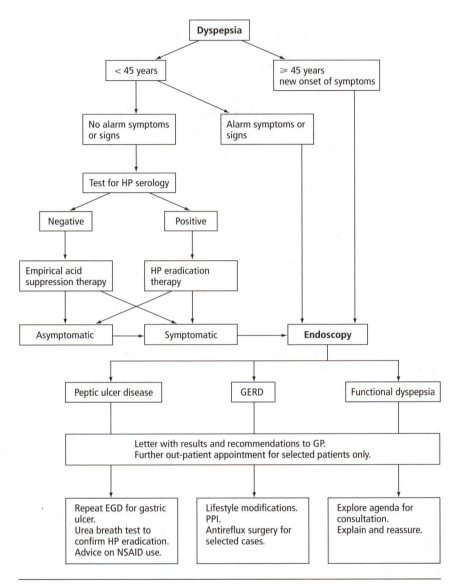

Figure 1.1. A 'test and treat' approach to dyspepsia

standard-dose PPI (choice of omeprazole, lansoprazole, pantoprazole, or rabeprazole) given twice daily for 7 days. Quadruple therapy with the inclusion of tripotassium dicitratobismuthate (bismuth chelate) 120 mg four times daily or an additional antibiotic (tetracycline 500 mg four times daily) to the above regime can be given for 2 weeks if eradication is not achieved with triple therapy.

Clinical studies and decision analysis models have shown that the benefit of the test-and-treat strategy is comparable to that of early endoscopy. In an unselected cohort of patients with dyspepsia, antibiotic therapy decreases dyspeptic symptoms by 14% in those patients with positive HP serology. However, one should take into account that only about 30–50% of unselected dyspeptic patients have positive HP serology. Studies comparing 'test and treat' with early endoscopy in a primary care setting showed comparable clinical outcome measures at 1 year including dyspepsia-free days, quality of life, or visits to the physician. The strategy decreases the demand for endoscopy, thereby producing substantial savings, at least in the short term. Further studies should clarify if a test-and-treat strategy has any superiority over early endoscopy in terms of patient satisfaction, healthcare utilization or long-term overall improvement in patient outcomes.

Empirical acid suppression

Guidelines of the AGA recommend a course of acid suppression therapy for HP-negative patients. Most patients with alarm symptoms do not have significant endoscopic abnormalities (low predictive value) but almost all patients with cancers will have alarm symptoms. An empirical trial of PPIs for 2–4 weeks would be expected to provide excellent symptomatic relief in the majority of patients with peptic ulceration or reflux esophagitis. Those who fail to respond to empirical treatment should then undergo endoscopy. The problem with this approach is mainly related to poor patient satisfaction. The patient may have had symptoms for some time and may have used over-the-counter remedies. It would be helpful to explore the patient's agenda for consultation, and explain the rationale of empirical acid suppressive therapy if appropriate.

Common diagnoses following investigations

Gastroesophageal reflux disease

The major pathophysiological event is the occurrence of transient lower esophageal sphincter relaxation. The relaxation is triggered by large meals, meals with high fat content, and lying down after eating. Reflux is exacerbated with certain food and drink such as chocolate and alcohol, and medications including bronchodilators, nitrates and calcium channel blockers.

Endoscopic evidence of esophagitis may be present in only 38–68% of patients with significant reflux symptoms. Patients should receive advice on lifestyle modifications such as weight loss or dietary changes. A course of a standard dose PPI for 4 weeks is effective in healing 95% of erosive esophagitis. Unfortunately, 80% of patients have been shown to develop recurrent esophagitis within 6 months if inadequate or no maintenance treatment is given. Symptomatic control for relapses may require use of intermittent courses of PPI, antacids, raft preparations, or H_2 antagonists. The new isomer of omeprazole,

Nexium®, is the only PPI at present that is licensed for use on an as-required basis. Continuous treatment with PPI (usually at lower dose) or H$_2$ antagonists may be beneficial for those with frequent, recurrent symptoms.

Anti-reflux surgery is usually considered for patients who are symptomatic or have recurrent strictures despite all medical treatment, or intolerance to PPI. It may also be performed if the patient wishes it, as long as they are fully informed of possible complications including dysphagia, bloating, difficulty in belching, and likely relapse of reflux symptoms. Preoperative esophageal manometry is usually performed together with a 24-h pH study: the former facilitates accurate placement of the pH electrode. These tests confirm the diagnosis of reflux and help rule out achalasia. The prevalence of esophageal dysmotility in GERD is approximately 30%, and symptomatic relief from anti-reflux surgery is not as good in these patients.

About 60% of surgically treated patients develop recurrent symptoms that require antisecretory medications when followed for 10 years after surgery. One of the predictors of successful surgery is a clinical response to medical therapy. A 24-h pH study is also helpful in the definitive diagnosis of GERD in symptomatic patients whose endoscopy is unremarkable.

Peptic ulcer disease

As many as 95% of duodenal ulcers are associated with HP and should receive a course of HP eradication therapy, in addition to a 4-week course of PPI. Repeat endoscopy is not necessary. A urea breath test should be considered to confirm eradication, especially in those with persistent or recurring symptoms. The yearly ulcer relapse rate in patients with persistent HP infection is about 80%, compared to less than 10% for those whose HP has been eradicated.

Infection with HP is associated with 70% of gastric ulcers. Biopsies should be taken from the ulcer for histology, and 8 weeks of treatment with PPI is recommended. Repeat endoscopy and biopsy is essential until epithelialization is completed.

When there is recurrence of symptoms, it is important to ensure clearance of HP infection and to discontinue NSAIDs. Recurrence of symptoms in an HP-negative patient not taking NSAIDs is an indication for repeating endoscopy.

Long-term antisecretory drug therapy is indicated for high-risk subgroups, including those with a history of complications, frequent recurrences, or refractory, giant or severely fibrosed ulcer.

Ulceration related to nonsteroidal anti-inflammatory drugs

About 5% of duodenal ulcers and 20–25% of gastric ulcers are related to the use of NSAIDs. Of patients taking NSAIDs, 2–4% develop ulcer-related complications within a year. These include GI hemorrhage, symptomatic ulcers, gastric outlet obstruction or gastroduodenal perforation. However, up to 40% of patients with NSAID-induced ulcers are asymptomatic and 60% of those who develop a hemorrhage have no prior symptoms. It is estimated that 2000 deaths due to NSAID-related side effects occur each year in the UK.

In patients who develop peptic ulcer-related complications while taking NSAIDs, these should be stopped or alternatively used concomitantly with gastro-protective agents. Misoprostol 200 µg four times daily has been shown in a large randomized trial (Misoprostol Ulcer Complications Outcomes Safety Assessment study) to reduce NSAIDs ulcer complications by 50%. However, side effects of diarrhea and abdominal cramps are common. Misoprostol and PPIs have been shown to be equally efficacious in reducing the rate of endoscopic ulcers. Newer NSAID agents such as nabumetone or cyclo-oxygenase 2 (COX-2) inhibitors induce fewer endoscopic ulcers and clinically important ulcer complications compared to standard NSAIDs in rheumatology patients. COX-2 inhibitors may be associated with fewer adverse upper GI tract symptoms than standard NSAIDs.

Recent guidelines published by the UK's National Institute for Clinical Excellence (NICE) on the use of COX-2 selective inhibitors in the treatment of osteoarthritis and rheumatoid arthritis recommended that these should be considered in preference to standard NSAIDs in those at risk of developing serious GI adverse events.

Box 1.1	Risk factors for GI complications with NSAID therapy
• Previous history of GI bleed, peptic ulceration or gastroduodenal perforation
• Age >65 years
• Presence of comorbidity, such as cardiovascular disease, renal or hepatic impairment, diabetes and hypertension
• Concurrent use of medications that increase likelihood of GI adverse events (e.g. steroids or anticoagulants)
• Prolonged use of maximum recommended doses of standard NSAIDs

Functional dyspepsia

FD or non-ulcer dyspepsia is defined as dyspeptic symptoms of at least 3 months' duration within the preceding 12 months, for which there is no structural or biochemical explanation. An upper GI endoscopy during a symptomatic period off acid suppressant therapy is essential to identify FD and exclude other structural diseases. The prevalence of FD is at least 40% of patients undergoing endoscopic and radiological evaluation for dyspepsia, but this may be an underestimate as it depends on patient selection.

Previous symptom-cluster classification of dyspepsia into ulcer-like, dysmotility-like or reflux-like dyspepsia has been shown to have little clinical utility. More recently, subgroup classification based on the predominant or most bothersome single symptom identified by the patient has been proposed. There is some evidence that suggests the latter may be more relevant and predictive of responses to treatment. This classification may also help to facilitate future research in this area.

Clinical studies of FD therapy is confounded by a high placebo response rate, with 20–60% of patients having symptom improvement on placebo. The studies of H_2 antagonists in FD have shown very variable results of treatment benefit but meta-analyses have suggested a therapeutic gain of up to 30% over placebo. This benefit appears spuriously large when compared with PPIs, which only showed a therapeutic gain of about 10% over placebo in clinical studies.

Psychological factors can often be identified in functional GI diseases, including FD. Increased lifetime psychiatric diagnosis is well documented in patients with functional GI disease and the psychiatric symptoms can sometimes predate GI ones. A psychological approach to therapy can be of benefit in some patients with FD. One study comparing psychotherapy (psychodynamic interpersonal therapy) with supportive therapy (as reassurance therapy) showed no difference in outcome at 12 months, but subgroup analysis suggested the treatment may be helpful for those with mild to moderate FD. Antidepressants, mostly tricyclic agents, have been successfully used for unexplained symptom syndromes such as functional bowel diseases and FD.

Helicobacter pylori in functional dyspepsia

Eradication of HP has been tested as a treatment for FD. Some studies showed the prevalence of HP to be higher in patients with FD than in healthy controls, which raised the possibility of a role of HP in FD symptoms. The results of studies looking for the benefit of HP eradication in FD have been mixed. A meta-analysis indicated a 9% benefit (relative risk reduction) in symptomatic improvement for treatment over placebo. Although the benefit appeared small, it was argued that if symptoms were sustained at 12 months, eradication would be cost-effective when compared to long-term PPIs. Another meta-analysis did not identify any significant difference in symptomatic improvement 1 year after treatment (eradication 35% vs. placebo 30%).

Between 4% and 21% of FD patients have an ulcer detected within 12 months. The potential benefit of preventing HP-positive FD patients from going on to develop peptic ulcer disease may favor the eradication strategy.

Although the eradication strategy may benefit a small number of HP-positive patients with FD, one needs to consider the cost, antibiotic-related side effects and development of resistant strains.

Dyspepsia clinics

There are two basic types of dyspepsia clinic. One approach involves a consultation in the outpatient department before organizing further tests such as endoscopy. The alternative approach is an open or direct access dyspepsia service offered by many endoscopy units. Patients undergo investigations including upper GI endoscopy or barium meal following referral from the GP, and only selected patients are given outpatient follow-up appointments.

There have been some studies supporting the first approach which suggested that patients initially seen by a gastroenterologist are more likely to undergo an endoscopy for appropriate indications, and the yield of endoscopy may be higher than those referred via the open access route. This approach also offers a chance to meet patients with a hidden agenda for consultation, who may be seeking the opportunity to discuss problems and/or any necessary procedures. This will increase patient satisfaction.

The drawback for the first approach is a significantly increased outpatient workload, which leads to a longer waiting time. The second approach avoids this pitfall, as follow-up appointments can be restricted to selected patients with abnormal investigations or specifically at the GP's request. The avoidance of a long waiting time for outpatient consultation before any investigation reduces patients' anxiety. Whether earlier diagnosis affects prognosis in patients who turn out to have GI malignancy remains to be established. When combined with written guidance to GPs on the 'test and treat' approach, this may add to the benefits of the investigations. One outcome study in general practice showed that open access gastroscopy is associated with rationalization of drug therapy, reduced consultations and a low hospital referral rate. In the presence of a safe and reliable mechanism for relaying the results and recommendations, GPs tend to be more satisfied with the second approach, which gives them more clinical autonomy.

An integrated option combining both approaches is the one-stop dyspepsia clinic. The concept of a one-stop approach has been practiced in several other specialties such as urology, surgery and ophthalmology. The essence of a one-stop service is that the patients are seen by medical staff, undergo investigations and are given a management plan all on the same day (see *Figure 1.2*). This has the obvious attraction of convenience for patients, especially those attending hospitals that cover a large geographical catchment area. In a study where a one-stop approach was used for open access referrals, this showed 14% of referrals to open access endoscopy were considered inappropriate and 24% of patients were asymptomatic when seen. Over a 1-year period, 25% of patients referred did not undergo endoscopy, with consequent financial savings.

Some reorganization of working practice and planning involving the radiology department may be necessary to implement a one-stop dyspepsia service. Our experience in Cornwall suggests this approach offers the highest satisfaction for patients and GPs alike.

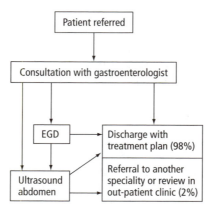

Figure 1.2. A 'one-stop' approach to dyspepsia

Further reading

British Society of Gastroenterology (1996) *Dyspepsia management guidelines. British Society of Gastroenterology Guidelines.*

Talley, N.J., Silverstein, M.D., Agreus, L., *et al.* (1998) AGA technical review: evaluation of dyspepsia. *Gastroenterology* **114**: 582–595.

Talley, N.J., Stanghellini, V., Heading, R.C., *et al.* (1999) Functional gastro-duodenal disorders. *Gut* **45**(suppl 2): II37–42.

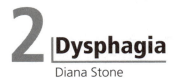

2 Dysphagia

Diana Stone

Introduction

Dysphagia is defined as a difficulty in swallowing. It often heralds significant esophageal pathology and the symptom of true dysphagia should always be investigated urgently. There are many causes of dysphagia (see *Box 2.1*) but in clinical practice the four most commonly encountered causes are:

- Peptic strictures
- Esophageal malignancy
- Esophageal dysmotility
- Achalasia

This chapter will concentrate on these four main causes and the setting up of a dysphagia clinic.

Box 2.1	Causes of dysphagia	
Oropharyngeal		**Esophageal**
Structural		*Mechanical*
Tumors		Tumor
Inflammation		Stricture
Radiation fibrosis		Web
Diverticula		Foreign body
Webs		Goiter
Cervical osteophytes		Large left atrium
Cervical tumors		Metastatic disease
Thyromegaly		
Motor		*Motility*
Stroke		Achalasia
Multiple sclerosis		Dysmotility
Motor neuron disease		Connective tissue disease
Extrapyramidal		Chagas disease
(e.g. Parkinson's)		
Guillain–Barré		*Others*
Myasthenia		Gastroesophageal reflux
Polymyositis		Esophagitis
Myotonic dystrophy		Esophageal ulcer

Management approach

History

The importance of good history taking is paramount in deciding the most appropriate investigations. Initially true dysphagia needs to be distinguished from globus and odynophagia (painful swallowing). It then needs to be decided whether the dysphagia is oropharyngeal or esophageal (see *Box 2.2*).

The length and pattern of the symptoms are also important features to elicit. Longstanding, intermittent dysphagia is more likely to be due to dysmotility or achalasia whereas continuous progressive symptoms are more suggestive of a mechanical obstruction. A short history of mechanical esophageal dysphagia with weight loss is carcinoma of the esophagus until proven otherwise. Whether the symptoms occur with liquids, solids or both should also be determined, as dysphagia for solids progressing to liquids is more common when the cause is mechanical.

Box 2.2	Distinguishing features of globus, esophageal and oropharyngeal dysphagia	
Oropharygeal	**Esophageal**	**Globus**
High dysphagia (at or above the sternal notch)	High or low dysphagia	No true dysphagia (lump in throat)
Symptoms immediately after swallowing	Symptoms delayed after swallowing	Symptoms often improved with swallowing
Choking and nasal regurgitation	No associated choking or regurgitation	No associated choking or regurgitation
May be unable to initiate swallow	Able to initiate swallow	Able to initiate swallow
May have features of underlying neurological disorder		May have underlying anxiety disorder

The past medical history can also give clues to the etiology. A history of reflux is found in 75% of patients with a benign peptic stricture. Associated chest pains are more common with achalasia and dysmotility. A past history of Barrett's metaplasia should alert the clinician to the possibility of esophageal adeno-carcinoma. In Barrett's esophagus there is a 2–3% lifetime risk of esophageal adenocarcinoma.

A detailed drug history should also be taken. Anticholinergics or neuroleptics such as phenothiazines can exacerbate dysphagia. The bisphosphonate, alen-dronate, can cause an esophageal stricture and obviously a history of ingestion of any caustic substances is important in this regard.

Any symptoms of aspiration, for example, cough, sputum, fever or shortness of breath should be sought and the clinician should be satisfied that oral intake is adequate.

Physical examination

A thorough examination to exclude any of the underlying causes of dysphagia should be undertaken. A full neurological examination is particularly important in the case of oropharyngeal dysphagia as signs of underlying disease may be present, for example, Parkinson's disease or cerebrovascular disease. Respiratory examination to exclude aspiration is also necessary and any evidence of metastatic disease such as supraclavicular lymph nodes or hepatomegaly should be sought.

The patients' nutritional state and hydration should be assessed to determine whether admission is needed for intravenous fluids/feeding whilst investigations and treatment are instituted.

Investigations (see *Box 2.3*)

In all cases routine laboratory tests should be carried out to assess hydration and nutritional status. A chest radiograph is important to look for any extrinsic

Box 2.3 | Investigations of dysphagia

All cases	Oropharyngeal	Esophageal
Full blood count	Direct laryngoscopy	Barium swallow
Urea and electrolytes	Video fluoroscopy	Endoscopy
Liver function tests		Esophageal manometry
Bone profile		Radionucleotide studies
Chest radiography		

causes of dysphagia and to exclude aspiration. In the case of oropharyngeal dysphagia, investigations to exclude the underlying cause should be carried out as dictated by clinical findings, for example, CT scan of head in the case of suspected cerebrovascular accident.

Patients with symptoms of high dysphagia should initially be assessed by barium swallow to exclude pharyngeal pouches, as endoscopy may be hazardous. The initial investigation for low esophageal dysphagia is more controversial. Some gastroenterologists prefer a barium swallow first as early strictures, proximal rings and webs, dysmotility and early achalasia may be missed at endoscopy. Others prefer endoscopy as the investigation of first choice, as subtle mucosal changes can easily be missed on barium radiology. Endoscopy also allows biopsies to be taken of any pathology encountered.

Esophageal manometry is the 'gold standard' for the investigation of dysmotility and achalasia but is not available in all centers. Radionucleotide studies, although less sensitive than manometry, can be of use in centers with limited access to the latter or in conjunction with manometry and pH studies in equivocal cases.

Dysphagia clinics

Open access dysphagia clinics have been set up in some centers to facilitate the rapid assessment of patients with dysphagia. An audit of 109 referrals by Wilkins *et al.* in 1984 revealed that 90 patients had true dysphagia. Of these 26% had a malignant stricture, 36% peptic stricture, 13% esophagitis, 7% motility disorder and 4% had other organic pathology. No abnormality was found in 14%.

When designing a specialized dysphagia clinic it is important to incorporate a mechanism for fast-tracking of patients with warning symptoms of esophageal neoplasia. 'Dysphagia' is a common symptom in the community. A recent audit in our unit discovered that 50% of patients who are referred by their GP with 'dysphagia' for a barium swallow have symptoms of globus or have had symptoms for months or years. It would clearly be inappropriate to set up a fast-track service for such patients.

Another consideration when designing a fast-track dysphagia service is whether patients should have upper GI endoscopy or a barium swallow first. Our

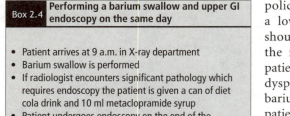

policy is that patients with a low esophageal dysphagia should have an endoscopy as the initial investigation and patients with a high esophageal dysphagia should have a barium swallow first. In those patients who have an abnormal barium swallow and require an endoscopy, this is performed on the same day by giving the patient a can of diet cola drink and 10 ml of metaclopramide syrup. This reliably clears all the barium from the upper GI tract within 3 hours.

The way the dysphagia clinic is being developed in our unit is summarized in *Figure 2.1.*

Peptic stricture

Peptic stricture usually occurs as a result of gastroesophageal reflux, particularly in the elderly. Of patients with peptic stricture, however, 25% will have had no

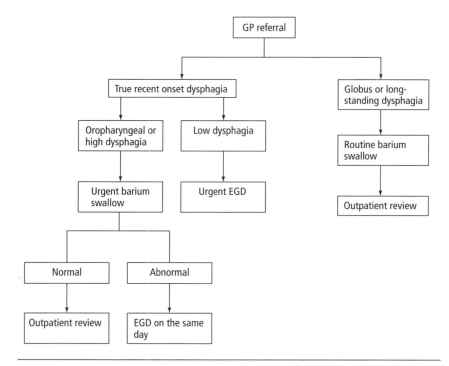

Figure 2.1. A 'one-stop' approach to dysphagia

prior symptoms of reflux. There is also an association between peptic stricture and NSAID ingestion.

Clinical presentation

Patients present with gradually increasing dysphagia, initially for solids but eventually for liquids. There will be a history of reflux symptoms in about 75% of cases. There can be weight loss but this is much less marked than in esophageal malignancy.

Investigations

A barium swallow will show a smooth tapering stricture in the lower esophagus. Endoscopy and biopsy are often performed to exclude malignancy.

Treatment

Most strictures are amenable to endoscopic dilatation under sedation. An esophageal lumen of less than 12 mm will cause dysphagia, so the aim is to dilate the stricture to between 12 and 18 mm. In the case of very tight strictures this may need to be done over a number of sessions.

Dilatation can be performed by balloon dilatation, by tapered plastic or rubber dilators or by metal olives. There is no data to suggest that any of these techniques are superior and the choice essentially lies with operator preference. The main complication of dilatation is perforation. This is far less common than in balloon dilatation for achalasia. Performing the dilatation under radiographic screening will reduce the risk of perforation, which should be less than 1%. Following successful dilatation, around 50% of patients will require redilatation within 1 year. One study showed that patients with no symptoms of heartburn and those with weight loss prior to the dilatation were more likely to need repeat procedures.

Recent studies have shown that high dose omeprazole (40 mg daily) after dilatation reduces the number of patients requiring repeat procedures and also prolongs the length of time between procedures in those that do require them. This advantage is not seen with H_2 antagonists and may be less marked with the other PPIs.

Surgery is reserved for cases that fail to respond to the above measures, and is seldom necessary. Fundoplication gastroplasty with pre- and postoperative dilatations is now the initial operation, with resection being reserved for fibrotic undilatable strictures and in patients where the gastroplasty fails.

Esophageal malignancy

The majority of esophageal tumors are either adenocarcinomas or squamous cell carcinomas. Both present in a similar fashion and both have a very poor prognosis. The incidence of adenocarcinoma is rising rapidly in the West for reasons that are not fully understood, and tends to occur in areas of Barrett's metaplasia. The risk factors for esophageal carcinoma are listed in *Box 2.5*. Squamous cell carcinoma has a strong geographical variation, with extremely high incidence in the Transkei in South Africa and across Northern China.

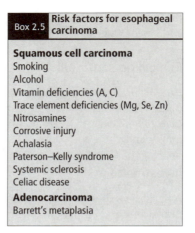

Clinical presentation

Both types of neoplasm present in the same way with a short history of progressive dysphagia, initially for solids and finally for liquids. There is often a profound weight loss and the patient can look extremely cachectic. Chest pain and odynophagia may be present and bleeding from the lesion may present as hematemesis, melena or anemia.

Investigations

A double-contrast barium swallow may show an irregular filling defect or a stricture. Endoscopy should always be performed for biopsy and brush cytology. The lesion at endoscopy can be anything from a whitish patch to a fungating tumor. A CT scan of the thorax and upper abdomen is necessary for staging. Endoscopic ultrasound (EUS) is the most sensitive investigation to detect local spread. EUS is superior to CT in assessing the depth of the tumor extension into the esophageal wall and in detecting local lymph node spread. A recent study of 50 patients compared staging at EUS to staging after surgery and histology. This showed EUS to be 92% accurate at T staging and 86% accurate at N staging (*Table 2.1*).

Table 2.1. TMN staging of esophageal carcinoma

Primary tumor (T)	Nodes (N)	Distant spread (M)
T1: Invading lamina propria/submucosa	N0: No nodes	M0: No metastases
T2: Invading muscularis propria	N1: Nodes	M1: Metastases
T3: Invading adventitia		
T4: Invading adjacent structures		

Treatment

Early carcinoma

The earlier stage the malignancy is detected, the better the potential outcome. Some early tumors (T1/T2) have as much as a 75% 5-year survival and much less invasive treatment such as endoscopic resection and photodynamic therapy can be offered.

Surgery

In order for the tumor to be potentially curable, it must be resectable (a third of cases) and the patient must be medically fit for the operation. In all, about 10% of esophageal malignancies are potentially curable. Some specialist centers have achieved a 60–80% 5-year survival in these patients, however these have been highly selected patients and a more realistic figure would be 35%. Studies have shown that for locally advanced adenocarcinoma, preoperative chemoradiation using fluorouracil, cisplatin and radiotherapy have increased the 3-year survival rates from 6% to 32%.

Radiotherapy

Some studies have suggested that, in particular for squamous cell carcinoma, radiotherapy can give a 5-year survival rate of 10%.

Palliation

The mainstay of palliation is to relieve the obstruction so the patient can tolerate a diet as near to normal as possible. Endoscopic dilatation may be helpful for short-term relief. A percutaneous gastrostomy (PEG) may be considered to maintain adequate nutritional intake, but the palliative procedure of choice is an expandable metal mesh stent. This achieves good symptom control in 80% of patients and has a relatively low incidence of complications compared to the old-fashioned semi-rigid plastic stent. Major complications are rare and perforation is relatively uncommon. Stent-related mortality, usually due to delayed GI bleed or aspiration pneumonia, is reported as less than 6%. Stent migration is seen in up to 30% of cases. Significant gastroesophageal reflux occurs in 10–20% of cases. Occasionally tumor overgrowth can block the stent. This can be treated with argon beam diathermy or by the placement of another stent, or by a combination of the two. The malignant stricture may be amenable to dilatation but this often needs repeating and there is a much higher perforation rate than with the dilatation of benign strictures. Radiotherapy in the form of external beam or brachytherapy may help achieve palliation. Alternatively, YAG photocoagulation is also useful but usually needs repeating although radiotherapy can prolong the interval between procedures. Alcohol injection (0.5–1 ml of ethanol) injected into multiple sites has also been used but is much less effective than other methods.

Achalasia

The word achalasia means 'failure to relax'. The condition is characterized by failure of both peristalsis and lower esophageal sphincter relaxation. This is due to degeneration and loss of ganglion cells in Auerbach's plexus. The inhibitory neurons are principally affected and there is a marked decrease in their chief neurotransmitter, nitric oxide, in the lower esophageal sphincter.

Clinical presentation

Achalasia is a progressive disorder generally occurring over the age of 40 years, although it is occasionally seen in younger patients. It often presents with a low dysphagia for solids, which is initially intermittent but eventually becomes constant. There may be associated chest pain that classically radiates through to the back and is increased by ingestion of cold liquids. The patient experiences weight loss, and regurgitation of retained esophageal contents especially at night may lead to aspiration and cough. Gastroesophageal reflux and halitosis are the other common complaints.

Investigations

Plain chest radiography shows a widened mediastinum with a fluid level and absence of the gastric bubble. A barium swallow classically reveals a dilated esophagus with the lower end tapered in a ' bird's beak' appearance. There is also failure of the lower esophageal sphincter relaxation after a food bolus, which can be detected by radiographic screening during the barium swallow examination. Endoscopy is always indicated as there is an increased incidence of squamous cell carcinoma in achalasia, and lower esophageal tumors can sometimes give the radiological appearance of achalasia (pseudo-achalasia).

The 'gold standard' investigation is esophageal manometry. This will reveal absent peristalsis in the lower esophageal muscle, failure of lower esophageal sphincter relaxation with swallowing and an increase in intraesophageal and basal sphincter pressure.

Treatment

The treatment options for achalasia include balloon dilatation, injection of botulinum toxin or surgical myotomy.

Dilatation is performed using a 30–40 French balloon dilator. There is no evidence as to the optimal pressure with which to inflate the balloon or for how long the balloon should be inflated. This usually relies on the operator's previous experience. Our unit's policy is to dilate at 15 psi (about 100 kPa) for 1 minute on two occasions. This is a very effective treatment with up to 65% of patients being dysphagia-free at 5 years. The possible side effects include perforation (3%) and symptomatic acid reflux. Patients should be admitted overnight and any suggestion of perforation (fever, chest pain, odynophagia, and surgical emphysema) should be investigated with a chest radiograph and water-soluble contrast swallow.

Botulinum A toxin–hemagglutinin complex when injected (total dose of 100 units of Botox®) around the lower esophageal sphincter (LOS) inhibits acetylcholine release from the nerve fibers. Initial results of this treatment are encouraging although most patients require more than one procedure. Patients over the age of 50 years tend to have a better result than younger patients. It has an advantage over dilatation in that there is a much lower incidence of perforation and this is now the treatment of choice in elderly and frail patients.

Surgical myomotomy is sometimes indicated in the young or when the above treatments have failed. The operative mortality however is 1%, and 10% of patients will develop significant reflux, for this reason a fundoplication is often performed simultaneously. Classically the operation is an open one via the abdomen or thorax, but more recently laparoscopic, thoracoscopic and endoscopic procedures are being introduced.

Esophageal dysmotility

Clinical presentation

The dysmotility disorders usually affect the lower two-thirds of the esophagus and present with an intermittent dysphagia and chest pain usually experienced with eating and at night.

Investigations

A barium swallow may show uncoordinated contractions, a corkscrew configuration, and an ineffective transport of barium and bolus. Endoscopy is usually normal although pronounced tertiary contractions may be seen. The investigation of choice is esophageal manometry, which may show abnormally prolonged or high amplitude contractions and an abnormally high basal sphincter pressure.

Treatment

Adequate treatment of this condition can be difficult. Many smooth muscle relaxants have been tried with variable success and a trial of nitrates and calcium channel antagonists may give symptomatic improvement. Treatment of any coexisting reflux may dramatically improve symptoms. Occasionally, in the presence of underlying psychiatric conditions, psychotropic drugs and behavior therapy may help.

If the above fail, dilatation or surgery may be contemplated. Balloon dilatation of the esophageal body with a 30 or 35 mm Rigiflex balloon, avoiding the lower esophageal sphincter, has been shown to improve symptoms in up to 50% of patients.

Further reading

Wilkinson, S.P. (1997) *Clinicians' Guide to Oesophageal Disease.* Chapman & Hall.

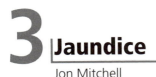

3 Jaundice

Jon Mitchell

Introduction

The acutely jaundiced patient is a common problem for the practicing gastro-enterologist. Rapid assessment, diagnosis and treatment are especially important in this group of patients as delays may result in significant morbidity and mortality. It is important to differentiate the patients with acute onset of jaundice from those with chronically deranged liver function tests (LFTs). This latter group can be more effectively investigated in a conventional outpatient setting and are covered in Chapter 7.

Traditionally, the acutely jaundiced patient has often been admitted directly to hospital as an emergency. This is often unnecessary as most can be safely assessed and managed on an outpatient basis. Depending on the local availability of outpatient clinics, radiology and endoscopy, it may be necessary to establish 'open-access' services where these patients can be rapidly assessed and appropriate management can be instigated without delay. An example of such a service is shown in *Figure 3.1*.

The aim of this chapter is to guide the clinician through the process of assessing the acutely jaundiced patient, from clinic organization to the appropriate investigations. It is not and does not purport to be a detailed text on the causes of jaundice and their subsequent management.

Setting up a jaundice service

The success of any service relies heavily on teamwork. All required medical, nursing and paramedical disciplines should be closely involved in the initial planning stage and in the subsequent running of the clinic.

Referral and access

Ease of access to the jaundice service for the referring clinician is pivotal to its success. The referral process should be straightforward and available both in and out of hours. A 24-hour answering service, fax machine or the use of electronic referrals may be appropriate depending on local resource availability. Referring clinicians should be encouraged, however, to provide the patient with a written referral on attendance. Vetting of referrals by a clinician should be avoided, if at all possible, as this will often introduce delays in the system, especially out of hours. Unless strict referral guidelines are established, however, the jaundice service will be susceptible to misuse. This may be in the form of inappropriate

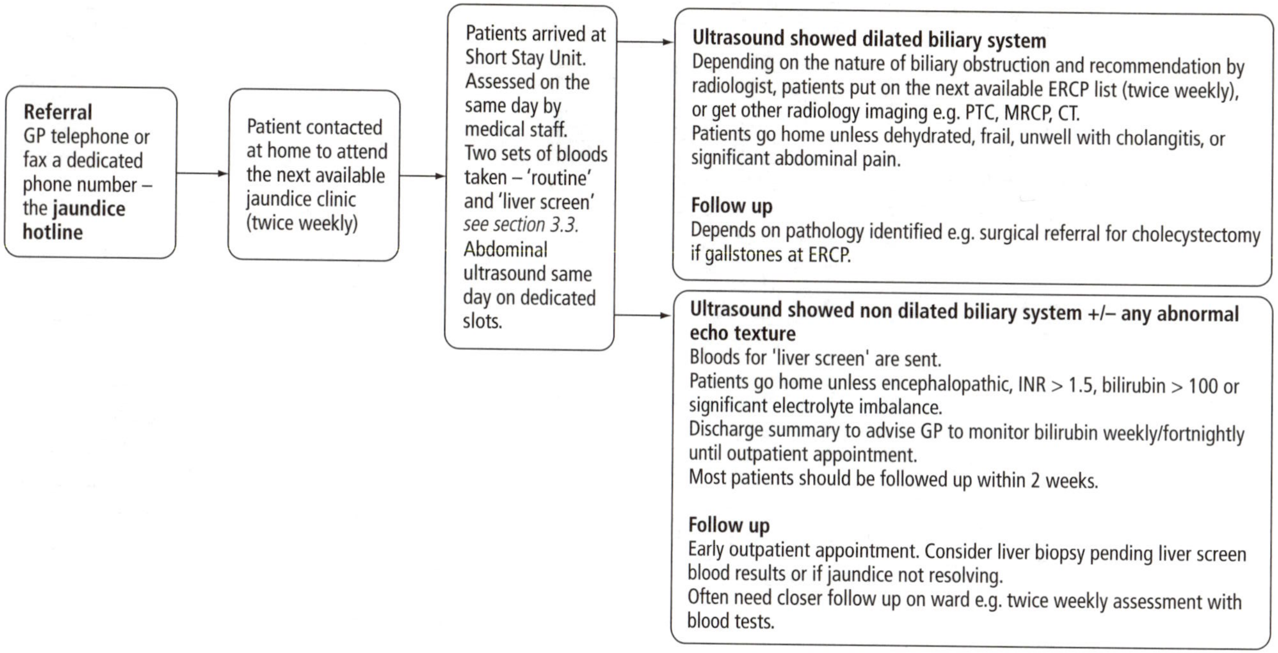

Referral
GP telephone or fax a dedicated phone number – the **jaundice hotline**

↓

Patient contacted at home to attend the next available jaundice clinic (twice weekly)

↓

Patients arrived at Short Stay Unit. Assessed on the same day by medical staff. Two sets of bloods taken – 'routine' and 'liver screen' *see section 3.3.* Abdominal ultrasound same day on dedicated slots.

→

Ultrasound showed dilated biliary system

Depending on the nature of biliary obstruction and recommendation by radiologist, patients put on the next available ERCP list (twice weekly), or get other radiology imaging e.g. PTC, MRCP, CT.
Patients go home unless dehydrated, frail, unwell with cholangitis, or significant abdominal pain.

Follow up
Depends on pathology identified e.g. surgical referral for cholecystectomy if gallstones at ERCP.

→

Ultrasound showed non dilated biliary system +/– any abnormal echo texture

Bloods for 'liver screen' are sent.
Patients go home unless encephalopathic, INR > 1.5, bilirubin > 100 or significant electrolyte imbalance.
Discharge summary to advise GP to monitor bilirubin weekly/fortnightly until outpatient appointment.
Most patients should be followed up within 2 weeks.

Follow up
Early outpatient appointment. Consider liver biopsy pending liver screen blood results or if jaundice not resolving.
Often need closer follow up on ward e.g. twice weekly assessment with blood tests.

Figure 3.1. A 'one-stop' approach to jaundice

referrals of patients with chronically abnormal LFTs. Examples of suggested guidelines for referral are:

- Patients must have *clinical* jaundice of not more than 4 weeks' duration
- The clinic is not designed to investigate patients with chronically deranged LFTs
- Referrals are by phone or fax and can be made at all times
- Although not essential, a written referral letter including all recent blood tests should be faxed or sent with the patient if at all possible
- The clinic is not designed as an alternative to the admission of acutely ill patients. Jaundiced patients may still require direct admission. If in doubt please discuss with a gastroenterologist or the physician on call. All patients with encephalopathy or evidence of sepsis should be admitted to hospital.

As with all such services, an efficient campaign to educate and publicize is integral to its success. This may take the form of a 'roadshow' to primary care practices and/or a flyer as written publicity.

Clinic frequency, location and staffing

Once the referral has been made, the patient is booked into the next available clinic. The timing, frequency and capacity of the clinic will depend partly on the local demand for such services. However, to prevent unacceptable delays between referral and attendance, clinics should be held at least twice per week. Experience with such services has shown that demand can soon outstrip supply. Auditing of pre-existing demand for such services will enable more efficient planning.

Clinic location will depend upon local resources. Outpatient departments, short-stay wards, medical admissions units and even endoscopy units may be appropriate. There must be enough space and privacy for venepuncture and a full examination, as well as discussion. It is important that the existing role of such areas is not compromised by the workload of a jaundice clinic or vice versa. Ideally, radiological services should be close at hand.

There is no reason why relatively junior medical staff cannot run an acute jaundice service as long as they receive education and written guidelines and are closely supervised by senior gastroenterologists. Guidelines for the investigation of this patient group are discussed at length later in this chapter. Senior staff should review all patients before decisions are made on further investigation (such as endoscopic retrograde cholangiopancreatography; ERCP), admission, discharge or follow-up. In our experience such a service can be an important part of the ongoing education of junior medical staff.

Skilled nursing staff can take on many aspects of the workload of an acute jaundice service, from venesection up to proforma-guided history taking. Integration of paramedical and nursing staff into the day-to-day running of the jaundice clinic will facilitate a high quality, multidisciplinary service.

The secretarial support required depends on the workload of the clinic. However, there is likely to be minimal extra clerical work required apart from written communications to the referring physician.

Radiological services

Ease of access to abdominal ultrasound performed by experienced radiologists is the key to success of any acute jaundice service. In fact such is the importance of this element, that any attempt to set up a jaundice clinic should only be contemplated as a joint venture between gastroenterologists and radiologists.

Flexibility of working is essential. The radiology department must have enough capacity to cope with demand, but also have the ability to fill 'slots' on quiet days with other work so as not to waste valuable scanning time.

The ultrasound service should preferably be run by experienced GI radiologists who can then be intimately involved with the decision-making process on further treatment.

Assessment of the acutely jaundiced patient

History

An accurate and detailed history is extremely important in the initial assessment of the jaundiced patient and is often useful in differentiating between biliary pathology and parenchymal liver disease. These findings can be recorded systematically on a form, enabling accurate record-keeping and providing guidelines for junior medical staff involved in the assessment process. An example of such a form, used by an established rapid access jaundice clinic, is shown in *Figure 3.2*.

Important features that need to be elicited in the history are shown in *Box 3.1*. It must be emphasized that these are in no way exhaustive, nor do they have a

Box 3.1	Important factors in the history of the acutely jaundiced patient
General	
Weight loss	malignancy
Pruritus	intra- or extra-hepatic cholestasis
Pain	common duct stones
Pale stools, dark urine	cholestasis, usually biliary
Fluctuation of jaundice	common duct stones
Prodromal symptoms	may be associated with viral hepatitis
Risk factors for liver disease	
Previous episodes of jaundice	
Blood transfusions	HBV, HCV
Intravenous drug use	HBV, HCV
Alcohol history	
Sexual history	HBV, HCV
Travel history	HAV, HBV, HEV, malaria
Drug history	include recent antibiotics, over-the-counter and herbal remedies, recreational such as MDMA
Contacts	
Environmental & food exposure	
Previous autoimmune disease	primary biliary cirrhosis, auto-immune hepatitis
Previous malignant disease	

Patient Label	Date Seen / /
	Seen by . . . .
	HO/SHO/SpR
	GP . . . .

Clinical Details

Transfusion?   Y/N
Foreign Travel?   Y/N
Prev. Jaundice?   Y/N

Medications (esp. recent antibiotics)

Warfarin?   Y/N

Examination

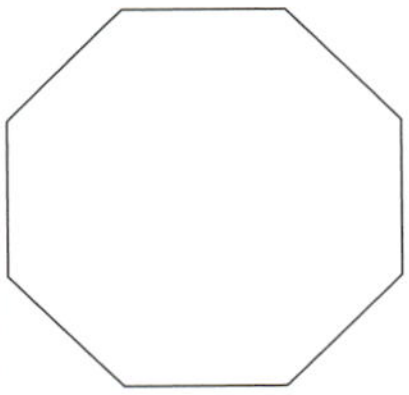

Jaundice Y/N

Pulse

BP   /

T   °C
S^1 S^2
Chest

Blood Results

Bilirubin   ALT

ALP   INR

Hb   WCC

Plt

Clinical Diagnosis

Ultrasound Result

Follow up

ERCP   Date   /   /
OP Review   Date   /   /

Comments

Figure 3.2. Clerking proforma for jaundice clinic

high degree of specificity. Jaundiced patients, like all others, constantly surprise and rarely conform to textbook criteria.

Physical examination

A full examination is mandatory. Combined with a well-taken history, the cause of jaundice can be predicted in a high proportion of cases before further investigations are performed.

General

Pulse, blood pressure and temperature should be noted. Look for signs of recent weight loss. Widespread lymphadenopathy may indicate Epstein–Barr viral infection (EBV) or even lymphoma. Scratch marks may indicate pruritus and therefore cholestasis even in a patient who denies such symptoms. Stigmata of chronic liver disease such as spider nevi, palmar erythema and gynecomastia should be sought. Tattoos, body piercings and needle marks may be relevant in cases of viral hepatitis.

Cardiovascular and respiratory

Look especially for a raised jugular venous pressure (JVP) and signs of right heart failure, which can occasionally cause hepatic congestion and jaundice, especially in the elderly. One of our patients who presented to the 'jaundice hotline' turned out to have an atrial myxoma!

Abdominal

Organomegaly should be sought and characterized. A palpable gallbladder suggests carcinoma of the head of the pancreas. Splenomegaly may indicate portal hypertension and therefore probable chronic liver disease, infections such as EBV or hematological complaints. Look further for evidence of chronic liver disease and ascites. A rectal examination should be performed if there is any suggestion of a neoplastic cause for the jaundice, rectal bleeding or recent change in bowel habit.

Neurological

Particular attention should be paid to the presence of encephalopathy as this necessitates admission in the acutely jaundiced patient. Look for cognitive impairment, constructional apraxia and liver flap. A reversed sleep pattern may suggest low-grade encephalopathy.

Initial investigations

Laboratory investigations

The availability of investigations will depend on the local laboratory policies. For clarity, these investigations are subdivided into general, virological, immuno-logical, metabolic and 'other'. In an acute jaundice clinic, it may be necessary to take enough blood for all investigations at presentation. There is, however, no point in requesting hepatitis virology, for example, on patients who are found subsequently to have a dilated biliary tree on ultrasound. Blood taken for such investigations can therefore be 'stored' and dispatched to the laboratory should ultrasound rule out an obstructive cause.

If an ultrasound examination has ruled out biliary obstruction or metastatic deposits, the following laboratory investigations will be indicated.

This list is, of course, not exhaustive. Investigation should be tailored to each individual patient. Instead, these could be thought of as guidelines for medical staff involved in the running of an acute jaundice service.

Ultrasound examination

A high-quality ultrasound examination is essential in the assessment of the acutely jaundiced patient. The primary role of ultrasound in this clinical setting is to detect biliary obstruction and provide further information as to its cause. The presence of biliary dilatation, gall bladder and ductal calculi, pancreatic

Box 3.3 Other investigations

1. Viral serology
Hepatitis B surface antigen *and*
Hepatitis B anti-core immunoglobulin M (IgM) if HBV suspected (more sensitive in acute infection)
Hepatitis A IgM
Epstein–Barr virus (+ monospot test if acute EBV suspected)
Hepatitis E IgM (recent travel to endemic areas; sporadic cases have been reported in the UK; rising IgG titres will confirm infection)
Note: Hepatitis C is a rare cause of acute jaundice. Testing for this virus is not a routine part of the investigation unless underlying chronic liver disease is suspected.

2. Immunology
Immunoglobulins (raised IgG in autoimmune hepatitis; raised IgA favors alcohol-induced injury)
Autoantibody profile (smooth muscle antibodies are positive in autoimmune hepatitis)
Note: Negative autoantibodies and immunoglobulins do not rule out autoimmune disease. Repeat at intervals if autoimmune hepatitis suspected.

3. Metabolic
Ferritin (acute phase reactant; may suggest underlying hemochromatosis)
Ceruloplasmin & copper studies (only in selected patients – a 70-year-old woman is unlikely to have Wilson's disease!)

4. Other
Alpha-fetoprotein (nonspecific elevation in chronic and acute liver disease; grossly elevated in hepatocellular carcinoma)
Hemolysis screen (not all jaundice is hepatological!)

tumors and hepatic metastases can all be established with high degrees of sensitivity. In addition, in cases of biliary obstruction, the radiologist can guide subsequent imaging or therapeutic intervention.

Although obstructive causes will account for the majority of presentations to an acute jaundice clinic (over 60% in our experience of such a service), ultrasound provides vital information in the diagnosis of parenchymal liver disease. Hepatic size and outline, the presence of fat and splenomegaly, may all provide information as to the presence of pre-existing liver disease. The presence of metastatic deposits and abdominal lymphadenopathy may be established. Doppler examination of the portal and hepatic veins may demonstrate the presence of portal hypertension or liver congestion and is essential to make the very important diagnosis of Budd–Chiari syndrome.

Following the ultrasound, close liaison with the radiologist will allow further investigations and therapeutic interventions to be planned. As has already been emphasized, this teamwork approach is essential to the success of the service.

Further investigations, admission and follow-up

The success of any rapid assessment service is determined by the availability of subsequent investigations, the ability to admit particularly sick patients directly from the clinic and easy access to rapid follow-up in the outpatient department. There is a little point in quickly establishing that a jaundiced patient has common bile duct obstruction secondary to gallstones, for instance, if ERCP to relieve the obstruction cannot then be performed for several weeks.

Obstructive jaundice

Decisions on further investigation in this patient group must be made with close liaison with the GI radiologist.

Early ERCP will be needed for many patients, especially those with choledocholithiasis and those with low common bile duct obstruction secondary to pancreatic head carcinoma. In the latter group, pancreatic computed tomography (CT) will also be required. The timing of this will depend upon local availability and whether the patient is felt to be a candidate for resection.

In patients with high common bile duct obstruction and especially in those with complex hilar lesions, percutaneous transhepatic cholangiography (PTC) may be a more appropriate procedure. Magnetic resonance cholangiopancreatography (MRCP) and EUS may be appropriate for some patients, either alone or in addition to other investigations.

Elderly or frail patients and those with evidence of cholangitis or dehydration should all be considered for direct admission to hospital.

Nonobstructive jaundice

This patient group presents several challenges to the rapid access jaundice clinic. Firstly, this is a much more heterogenous group presenting significant diagnostic and management difficulties. An experienced gastroenterologist or hepatologist, therefore, should be consulted about all these patients.

Secondly, although many of these patients will be suitable for outpatient follow-up, significant numbers will require direct admission to the ward and the remainder may warrant extremely close follow-up with regular blood tests every few days initially. For the latter group, flexibility of working and a team approach will be essential as it may not be possible or desirable to arrange follow-up in official outpatient clinics. Further blood checks may be necessary, for instance, on the ward.

As a rule all patients with encephalopathy and most with evidence of significant synthetic hepatic dysfunction (bilirubin > 100 or INR > 1.5) should be admitted directly for further investigation and management.

Communication and correspondence

The initial assessment of each jaundiced patient should be communicated back to the referring physician immediately. This may take the form of a copy of the clerking sheet. A more formal report detailing final diagnosis, further investigations and clinical course can follow at a later date. Modern services require a modern approach to effective communication and use of the Internet would seem an ideal method of providing instantaneous feedback.

Opportunities also arise for patient information in this setting (see Chapter 18). Patient information leaflets cover general hepatological issues and also function as an aid to fully informed consent for procedures such as ERCP. The provision of these leaflets and liaison with specialist hepatological and drug and alcohol nurses will aid the development of a truly integrated jaundice clinic as part of a multi-disciplinary approach to clinical gastroenterology.

The jaundice hotline: our experience

In 1998 the jaundice hotline was established in our hospital, employing the principles outlined in this chapter. The hospital is an 850-bed district general hospital and serves a population of approximately 400 000 patients spread over a very large geographical area.

On average the jaundice hotline sees 160 patients per year. There are two 'jaundice hotline' clinics per week. On average, once patients have seen their GP, they wait 2.5 days to be seen by the service. Patients who have an obstructed biliary system on ultrasound then wait an average 6 days for their ERCP. The diagnoses of the patients seen are shown in *Figure 3.3*. This service has saved approximately 800 inpatient bed-days per year and has been very well received by patients and GPs. The only cost of setting up this service was the purchase of the answerphone, to take referrals out of office hours.

In addition to these obvious advantages, establishing and running the jaundice hotline has promoted major improvements in teamwork and multi-disciplinary working in the GI unit.

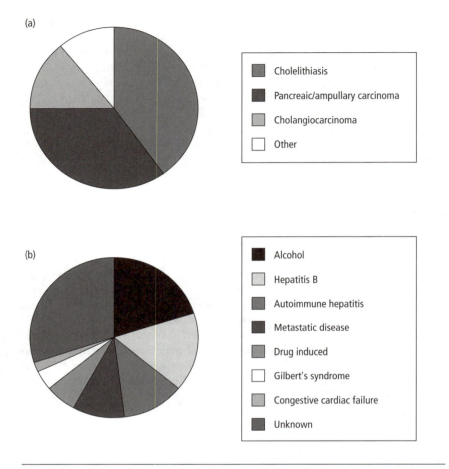

(a)

	Cholelithiasis
	Pancreaic/ampullary carcinoma
	Cholangiocarcinoma
	Other

(b)

	Alcohol
	Hepatitis B
	Autoimmune hepatitis
	Metastatic disease
	Drug induced
	Gilbert's syndrome
	Congestive cardiac failure
	Unknown

Figure 3.3. **Diagnoses from 107 patients seen in a jaundice clinic in a large general hospital. Divided into (a) obstructive Jaundice (*n*=62) and (b) non-obstructive jaundice (*n*=45)**

Further reading

Mitchell, J., Hussaini, S.H., and Dalton, H.R. (2000) The Jaundice Hot-line: a lesson in health service reorganisation. *Remedy* **8**: 16.

Mitchell, J., Hussaini, S.H., McGovern, D., Farrow, R., Maskell, G., and Dalton, H. (2002) Rapid assessment of the jaundiced patient: the Jaundice Hot-line. *Brit. Med. J.* **325**: 213–215.

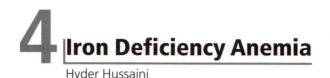

4 Iron Deficiency Anemia

Hyder Hussaini

Introduction

Iron deficiency anemia (IDA) accounts for up to 13% of GI referrals to the outpatient clinic. In patients over the age of 40, IDA with no associated symptoms may be indicative of occult gastric or colonic neoplasia or disorders such as celiac disease. To minimize patients' inconvenience and ensure early assessment, a one-stop approach to the investigation of patients with IDA can be used with clinical assessment and investigation on the same visit to the outpatient department.

Referral to one-stop iron deficiency clinic

All patients with proven biochemical iron deficiency (low ferritin or compatible iron studies) are suitable for referral to the iron deficiency clinic (see *Table 4.1*). Using these criteria patients do not need to be clinically anemic to undergo further investigation. We believe that this is logical since patients will manifest iron deficiency before anemia. The underlying cause for iron deficiency is likely to be the same in this cohort of patients, although there is no data from clinical studies to support this hypothesis. However, priority is given to patients with anemia – most of the patients seen in the clinic are or have been anemic.

Table 4.1. Criteria for iron deficiency

Ferritin	$< 12 \ \mu g \ dl^{-1}$
Reduced serum iron	$< 8.8 \ \mu mol \ l^{-1}$
Raised transferrin	$> 3.2 \ g \ l^{-1}$
Reduced iron saturation	< 16

Symptomatic patients with IDA are usually investigated through the conventional outpatient clinic, if IDA was determined after GP referral. Patients younger than 40 years who are asymptomatic with IDA are screened for celiac disease by checking endomysial antibodies (EMAB) and serum IgA (since EMAB can be falsely negative in IgA deficiency) prior to attending the iron deficiency clinic. Premenopausal women, with no GI symptoms and negative EMAB are usually seen in the conventional outpatient clinic, since this cohort seldom need endoscopic investigation.

Anemia Clinic

Hospital No. _____
Name _____
Age _____

Diagnosis	Y/N		Y/N
Anemia incidental finding		Anemia symptomatic	
		Dyspnoea	
		Lethargy	
		Others	

GI symptoms	Y/N	Non GI factors	Y/N
Dysphagia		Regular blood donor	
Vomiting/hematemesis		Vegetarian	
Weight loss		Frank hematuria	
Abdominal pain		Menorrhagia	
Chronic diarrhea (> 3 weeks)		brief details	
Melena			
Fresh bleeding per rectum			

Past history		Drug History	Y/N
Previous anemia episode(s)	Y/N	Aspirin	
Approximate date/year		NSAIDs	
		Long term steroids	
Previous investigation(s)	Y/N	Warfarin	
Approximate date/year			
brief details		Family History	Y/N
		Upper GI malignancy	
		Lower GI malignancy	
Previous GI surgery(s)	Y/N	Hemorrhagic telangiectasia	
Approximate date/year		Hematological disorders	
brief details		brief details	

Examinations

Urine dipsticks	

Clinical anemia	Y/N	Jaundice	Y/N
Lymphadenopathy	Y/N	Oral telangiectasia	Y/N
Abdominal mass	Y/N		
Description			

Recent blood tests

Approximate date done		Iron studies	
Hb		Ferritin	
MCV		Iron	
		Transferrin	
		Transferrin saturation	

Figure 4.1. IDA clinic proforma

Clinical assessment

Patients who fulfill criteria for referral to the clinic are sent a standard letter containing an appointment date and time, information about the clinic and the investigations that may be required. In patients over 40 years old, full bowel preparation is given since they will invariably need colonic investigation. All patients are instructed to fast beforehand since endoscopy may be required.

The iron deficiency clinic requires an endoscopist and additional doctor to clinically assess the patient before endoscopy. We use a standard proforma form (see *Figure 4.1*) which includes questions regarding upper and lower GI symptoms, concomitant drug therapy including aspirin and NSAIDs, and family history of GI cancer, telangectasia or disorders such as sideroblastic anemia. Although dietary intake is assessed and may be the cause for iron deficiency, the presence of poor intake does not preclude further investigation. Clinical examination for telangectasia and abdominal masses is performed together with urinalysis for blood and protein. This initial assessment leads to further investigation as outlined below, which differs depending on the age, symptoms and sex of the patient. Patients with significant comorbid disease or advanced age should be only investigated if the results of investigation would alter future management. In these cases the need for further investigation should be carefully discussed with the patient and relatives.

Investigations (see *Figure 4.2*)

Asymptomatic patients aged 40 years and over

In patients over the age of 40, both upper and lower GI investigation is routinely performed since dual pathology in the upper and lower GI tract is found in 10–15% of patients. Patients undergo gastroscopy with small bowel biopsy followed by colonoscopy. Alternatives to colonoscopy are a combination of flexible sigmoidoscopy with carbon dioxide insufflation followed by double-contrast barium enema or CT of the colon. CT of the colon is performed for patients over 80 years old, those few patients who are too frail to undergo colonoscopy or those who have incomplete colonoscopic investigation. Colonoscopy is preferred to barium contrast studies since angiodysplastic lesions can be visualized and colonic biopsies can be taken. Small bowel biopsy is mandatory since celiac disease may be present in 2–3% of patients.

Asymptomatic patients younger than 40 years

All patients with positive EMAB or IgA deficiency undergo upper GI endoscopy with small bowel biopsy to confirm or refute the diagnosis of celiac disease.

Asymptomatic young patients with a strong family history of colon cancer (two first-degree relatives or one first-degree relative under the age of 45),

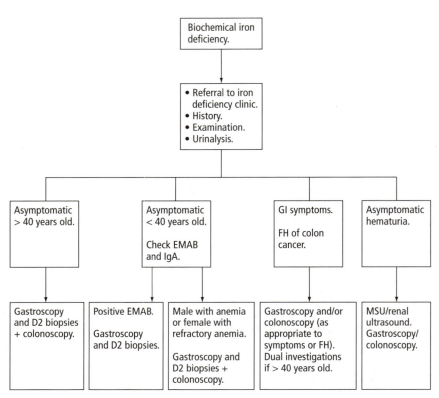

Figure 4.2. **Management of iron deficiency**

persistent anemia despite treatment with iron, or recurrent anemia should undergo colonoscopy and gastroscopy.

In male patients with anemia (hemoglobin < 11.5 g dl^{-1}) we currently advise initial gastroscopy, with a view to colonoscopy if no significant pathology is found. There is no data regarding the incidence of significant pathology in healthy males with asymptomatic anemia, thus dual investigation at the same session is seldom performed.

In view of the fact that IDA is common (5–10%) in premenopausal women, if patients are asymptomatic and are negative for EMAB with a normal IgA, then no further investigation is performed. Investigations can be considered when anemia is refractory to iron treatment.

Symptomatic patients

The initial endoscopic investigation is directed to the predominant symptom complex, for example, those with dyspeptic symptoms undergo gastroscopy. In patients over age 40, if the initial investigation is normal or reveals no major cause for anemia, then colonoscopy or gastroscopy as appropriate is performed.

Treatment

The underlying cause for anemia should be treated if found at gastroscopy or colonoscopy. Oral iron, usually ferrous sulphate (200 mg three times daily), will increase the hemoglobin by 2 g dl^{-1} over 3–4 weeks. Iron supplementation is recommended for a further 3 months after normalization of hemoglobin to replenish iron stores. Inpatients intolerant of more than two different oral iron supplements (including ferrous gluconate and fumarate) can be treated with parenteral iron therapy. For parenteral replacement, the total iron load is calculated and the patient can be admitted to a day case unit for a series of intravenous iron infusions. The risk of anaphylaxis with the modern parenteral iron therapies is minimal. We do not use intramuscular iron replacement, as this is very painful for the patient.

Normal gastroscopy and lower gastrointestinal investigations

Most patients with normal results from gastroscopy, duodenal biopsies and colonic investigations can be discharged to their GP. We ask the GP to insure that patients complete a 3-month course of iron treatment once the hemoglobin has returned to normal and to check the full blood count at 3-monthly intervals for 1 year after finishing iron treatment. If the anemia recurs then we ask for patients to be restarted on iron and referred for further assessment.

In patients aged between 40 and 60 years with normal results from gastroscopy, duodenal biopsies and colonoscopy, barium examination of the small bowel is performed to look for small bowel tumors, which rarely occur in this age group, and Crohn's disease. In older patients no further investigation is routinely performed.

Recurrent anemia

It is uncommon for anemia to recur in patients who have had normal results from gastroscopy, duodenal biopsies and colonic investigations. We initially treat patients with recurrent anemia with long-term iron supplementation. If this is ineffective and the patient becomes transfusion-dependent, then enteroscopy and small bowel radiology is performed. 'On table' endoscopy at laparotomy or laparoscopically assisted is useful in those patients with undiagnosed recurrent transfusion-dependent anemia. In the absence of overt bleeding, mesenteric angiography is unhelpful. Fecal occult blood testing is nonspecific and thus of little use in the management of IDA.

Asymptomatic hematuria with iron deficiency anemia

Renal tract tumors can occasionally present with IDA. Thus in addition to gastroscopy and colonoscopy, as clinically indicated, asymptomatic patients with hematuria should provide urine samples for microscopy and culture and undergo renal/pelvic ultrasound.

Summary

The iron deficiency clinic provides rapid, convenient access for patients to undergo clinical assessment and relevant investigation in a single visit. The clinic is predominantly for the rapid assessment of those patients at greatest risk of gastric and colorectal cancer. In general gastroscopy, duodenal biopsy and colonic investigation are sufficient to exclude major pathology. Further investigation is performed in younger patients with unexplained IDA and in those whose anemia does not respond to treatment with iron.

Further reading

Goddard, A.F., McIntyre, A.S. and Scott, B.B. (2000) *Guidelines for the Management of Iron Deficiency Anaemia.* British Society of Gastroenterology.

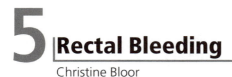

5 | Rectal Bleeding

Christine Bloor

Introduction

Patients who present with symptoms of colon cancer, such as rectal bleeding, change in bowel habit or IDA, may require investigation with a combination of flexible sigmoidoscopy and barium enema. With innovative planning and close collaboration between the endoscopy unit and the radiology department, it is possible to facilitate a one-stop service, which provides 'fast track' diagnosis and allows the patient to undergo both procedures on the same day.

In many centers, flexible sigmoidoscopy is carried out by nurse practitioners and barium enemas by specialist radiographers. Our local experience has been to train a clinical specialist radiographer, experienced in performing barium enemas, to carry out flexible sigmoidoscopy, which has resulted in a radiographer-led one-stop flexible sigmoidoscopy and barium enema service.

Setting up a training program for the endoscopist

Background

The growing demands for endoscopy services within the UK combined with the limited number of trained endoscopists, has resulted in the development of skills mix in this area. Flexible sigmoidoscopy is now routinely carried out by endoscopy nurses or colorectal nurse practitioners and there are a number of specialist courses to support this development. There is currently no training program available for radiographers wishing to perform endoscopic procedures. This resulted in the local development of a radiographer-focused flexible sigmoidoscopy training program.

Program design

The program was written by a consultant gastroenterologist and approved by the GI team and the hospital trust board. The course was constructed around a framework of practical and clinical skills delivered via an integrated training program. The content was designed to meet the learning needs of the individual, using adult learning principles to build on the learner's prior knowledge. It involved self-directed study and a process of personal and professional reflection. The trainee was also required to keep a logbook of training and experiences.

Training took place during two endoscopy sessions per week, with a consultant gastroenterologist and a consultant radiologist. The program encompassed social, professional, ethical and legal issues, which were explored contextually through discussion around individual clinical cases. Technical skills training was staged, structured and broken down into elements, with a logical progression from one to the next (see *Box 5.1*).

It began with the radiographer directly observing an experienced endoscopist performing flexible sigmoidoscopies. The radiographer practiced endoscopic control *in vitro* to become familiar with the controls and movements of the endoscope. This part (stage one) of the training program also allowed the radiographer time and opportunity to become familiar with the endoscopy unit and to integrate into the team.

Box 5.1	Technical skills training stages

Stage one: Observe 25 procedures
Aims
- Observe procedures
- Become familiar with unit
- Endoscopic control *in vitro*

Stage two: Perform 40 withdrawals
Aims
- Handle endoscope *in vivo*
- Knowledge of mucosal appearances
- Take biopsies

Stage three: Perform 85 full procedures
Aims
- Competent at safe insertion
- Identify pathologies
- Write reports
- Develop communication skills
- Decision-making

The next part (stage two) of the program involved the radiographer handling the endoscope *in vivo*, by withdrawing the endoscope after it had been advanced into the colon by the trainer. The radiographer then began to distinguish between normal and abnormal mucosa, identify pathologies and take biopsies. After endoscope withdrawal had been successfully achieved in 40 patients, the radiographer then progressed to performing full procedures.

During the next phase of the training program (stage three) the radiographer became competent at performing safe insertion and accurately identifying pathologies. The radiographer began taking responsibility for making decisions on clinical and practical aspects of the endoscopic procedure, which included writing and issuing the report. The radiographer was also encouraged to develop communication skills to obtain the patient's consent and discuss the endoscopic findings, within a safe and supervised environment. The radiographer developed professional and social communication within the endoscopy team, to become an accepted and credible member of the unit. After 85 full procedures had been completed and an accepted level of competency had been reached, a formal assessment was carried out before independent practice could begin.

Assessment (see also Chapter 19)

A formal, written assessment was carried out by an experienced GI endoscopist, who had not taken part in the endoscopy training program. The assessment was based on the direct observation of an endoscopy list. The assessment criteria included consent, endoscope control, recognition of normal and abnormal mucosal appearances, report writing and communication skills. In addition the radiographer and the assessor discussed each clinical case including the indications for performing the endoscopy and the possible alternatives. After a successful assessment the radiographer commenced independent endoscopic practice. After a period of 6 months the assessment was repeated in order to monitor progress, and it is envisaged that this process will be repeated annually as part of the clinical governance process. The radiographer also takes part in a regular appraisal program to support this new area of practice. This allows the discussion of clinical and professional issues and ensures continuing professional development and regular audit within this new community of practice.

Rectal bleeding clinics

Organization of a one-stop rectal bleeding service

The radiographer undertakes a flexible sigmoidoscopy list on two mornings per week with a maximum of seven patients per list. As many as nine patients per week can take part in the one-stop service and undergo a flexible sigmoidoscopy followed by a double-contrast barium enema. The majority of patients will have both procedures performed by the radiographer. The patients attend the endoscopy unit in the morning and those with an early appointment will have the barium enema that morning and those with a later appointment will have it in the afternoon. Carbon dioxide is used as the gas insufflating agent for flexible sigmoidoscopy, allowing the time between the two procedures to be kept to a minimum.

The success and efficient organization of this service depends on a collaborative working relationship between the endoscopy unit and the radiology department at all levels. Protected barium enema appointment slots are made available to coincide with the flexible sigmoidoscopy session, and fixed appointment times are given to each patient for both examinations.

The barium enema referral is checked by a consultant radiologist prior to the appointment being issued. Particular attention is given to the patient's age, mobility and general health. The barium enema examination requires the patient to be reasonably mobile. If the patient has poor mobility or a medical condition that precludes them from undertaking the examination, then appropriate alternative imaging can be arranged for the same day, for example, CT colon, CT colonography or colonoscopy.

Selection of patients

Patients are selected for the one-stop clinic from a number of different referral pathways. Many of the patients who attend have been referred by their GP with symptoms suspicious of colon cancer via the urgent '2-week wait' system. Attending the one-stop clinic insures that the patient undergoes the relevant diagnostic procedures before the consultant sees them, and that all results, including histopathology, are available at the patient's first outpatient clinic attendance. Patients that are referred to the one-stop clinic with IDA and symptoms of dyspepsia will undergo an upper GI endoscopy and duodenal biopsies as well as a flexible sigmoidoscopy and barium enema.

The endoscopy unit secretary takes responsibility for the administrative side of the service by both organizing appointments and liasing with the radiology department. The appointments for endoscopy and radiology are sent out together, including the bowel preparation and all the relevant patient information leaflets. The secretary also provides one point of contact for patients and staff and ensures a continuous level of service.

Use of carbon dioxide

Room air has been traditionally used as the insufflating agent for flexible sigmoidoscopy and barium enema. However, several studies have shown that the abdominal distention and post-procedural pain experienced by patients after barium enema or colonoscopy is significantly reduced if carbon dioxide is used. This is due to the rapid absorption of carbon dioxide through the wall of the large bowel, which is then carried to the lungs and exhaled. The technical quality of the barium enema study is reliant on good mucosal coating and the patient's ability and willingness to cooperate. The use of carbon dioxide as an insufflating agent for flexible sigmoidoscopy prior to barium enema ensures there is minimal residual gas in the colon, and allows for good mucosal coating. The pain and discomfort experienced by the patient between procedures is reduced significantly and the time gap between the two procedures can be reduced to as little as 1 hour.

It is possible to fit a carbon dioxide button, in the usual air button position, to most modern endoscopes and a low pressure, metered flow, carbon dioxide delivery system is now readily available at a reasonable price, making the use of carbon dioxide accessible to most units.

Bowel preparation

Good bowel preparation is essential in obtaining an optimal examination of the colon both endoscopically and radiologically, and as both procedures are being performed on the same day, the entire colon must be free from fecal residue and excess fluid. Inadequate bowel preparation can result in poor endoscopic views of the mucosa and on barium enema it may be difficult to distinguish between fecal residue and pathology. Excess fluid can be removed through the suction channel of the endoscope but any remaining fluid will result in poor barium coating of the colon, and a reduction in diagnostic accuracy.

There are a number of bowel cleansing agents available and the chosen preparation should combine efficacy with tolerance by the patient. It is unlikely that any single bowel preparation will suit all patients, and it is advisable to have alternatives available. The most commonly used preparations are Picolax® (sodium picosulphate), Fleet Phospha-Soda®, Klean Prep® and Citramag®. Picolax® is widely used in preparing the colon for diagnostic investigations and surgery. In our experience it has been found to yield good results in terms of the cleanliness of the colon and barium coating, it is also well tolerated by most patients.

A clear fluid diet is recommended for 24 hours before the combined procedures. If this is not possible then patients must restrict their diet to exclude high-fiber foods. Patients who suffer from diabetes may find a fluid-only diet a particular problem. We therefore provide patients with a contact telephone number for a diabetic nurse specialist or endoscopy nurse who can give accurate advice on the management of diet and diabetic drugs. Morning barium enema slots are reserved for patients with diabetes in order that the patient can recommence hypoglycemic medication with a midday meal.

Summary

The radiographer-led one-stop service provides a safe, cost-effective and efficient 'fast-track' diagnostic service for patients with suspected cancer. It is more convenient for patients as they have to endure only one bowel preparation and one trip to the hospital. It also ensures that the patient receives continuity of care and service throughout both departments.

This innovative approach to skills mix has encouraged and enhanced multidisciplinary teamwork between the radiology department and the endoscopy unit. The radiographer now carries out two complementary practices and works as an advanced diagnostic practitioner within the GI team, providing a link between all disciplines and all grades.

The success of the service relies on the cooperation and collaboration of staff at all levels within both units. As a result working relationships have been enhanced and are now more flexible.

Further reading

Cancer Services Collaborative (2001) *Bowel Cancer: Service Improvement Guide.* NHS Modernising agency. www.nhs.uk/npat
Cancer Services Collaborative (2001) *Radiology: Service Improvement Guide.* NHS Modernising Agency. www.nhs.uk/npat

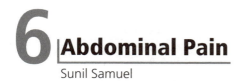

6 Abdominal Pain

Sunil Samuel

Introduction

Abdominal pain is one of the commonest symptoms that gastroenterologists encounter both in outpatients and inpatients. This can sometimes provide a major diagnostic challenge, particularly in patients who are unable to give a good history. However, a good history, thorough examination and a basic understanding of typical patterns and clinical presentations of common diseases should help in making a diagnosis in most cases.

Abdominal pain can be categorized as visceral, parietal or referred. Visceral pain is dull and aching in character. It is poorly localized and is usually secondary to distention or spasm of a hollow viscus. Parietal pain is sharp and well localized and arises from irritation of the parietal peritoneum. Referred pain is the perception of pain at a site distant from the origin of the stimulus. One possible explanation for this is that the visceral and the somatic afferent nerve fibers share a common pathway at the level of the cord, which is the spinothalamic tract. The brain tends to associate the stimulation more with a somatic source rather than visceral. This type of pain is characteristically aching and perceived to be near the surface of the body. For example, referred pain from gallstones is sometimes perceived in the right shoulder because some of the afferent pain fibers run in the right phrenic nerve (C3–5).

Pain physiology

It is important to have a basic understanding of some of the physiological factors that cause abdominal pain.

The main visceral pain receptors in the abdomen respond to mechanical and chemical stimuli. The mechanical stimuli perceived are stretch, distention, contraction, compression and torsion. The chemical stimuli include substance P, bradykinin, serotonin, and prostaglandins. These receptors are located on the serosal surfaces, within the mesentery and within the walls of the hollow viscera.

Gut-related visceral pain is usually perceived in the midline because of bilateral symmetric innervation, except for pains originating from the gallbladder and the ascending and descending colon. Pain originating from other intra-abdominal organs generally tends to be unilateral.

The perception of visceral pain corresponds to the spinal segments where the visceral afferent nerve fibers enter the spinal cord. For instance, distention of small bowel causes discomfort in the periumbilical area (T8–L1). *Table 6.1* shows some of the common spinal segments where visceral pain is perceived.

Table 6.1. Dermatomal perception of visceral pain

Abdominal organs	Site of pain	Dermatomes
Stomach	Epigastrium	T6–T10
Small bowel	Umbilical	T9–T10
Gallbladder	Epigastrium	T7–T9
Pancreas	Epigastrium	T6–T10
Colon up to splenic flexure	Umbilical	T11–L1
Colon from splenic flexure	Hypogastrium	L1–L2
Testis and ovary	Umbilical	T10–T11

Management approach to a patient with abdominal pain

History

As in most disciplines in clinical medicine, the history will give the most important clues to the cause of abdominal pain. In most settings 90% of the information regarding the pain is gleaned from the history and only 10% from clinical examination. It is important to characterize the specific features of the pain.

Character

The character of the pain helps to a certain extent to identify the pathology: the 'burning' or 'gnawing' type of pain is typical of gastro-esophageal reflux and peptic ulcer; 'colicky' pain is seen in gastroenteritis or intestinal or biliary obstruction.

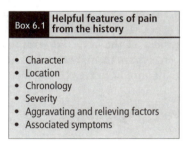

Box 6.1 Helpful features of pain from the history

- Character
- Location
- Chronology
- Severity
- Aggravating and relieving factors
- Associated symptoms

Location

Location of the pain strongly suggests its origin. For each organ the pain is usually most severe at its primary site and is variably perceived at secondary sites (also called radiation or projection of pain). For example, when the primary site of pain is in the epigastrium the source usually is the stomach, duodenum and pancreas and this is frequently projected to the midline over the lumbar spine, which is the secondary site of pain. *Table 6.2* gives some of the differential diagnoses for different primary sites of pain.

Chronology

Chronology in the form of date of onset and circumstances surrounding the beginning of abdominal pain is important. For example, abdominal pain due to chronic pancreatitis can be longstanding and could have started following abdominal trauma that occurred in an accident where the pancreatic injury was

Table 6.2. Causes of abdominal pain by location

Right upper quadrant	Epigastric	Left upper quadrant
Cholecystitis	Peptic ulcer disease	Splenic infarct
Cholangitis	Reflux disease	Gastric ulcer
Subdiaphragmatic abscess	Pancreatitis	Pancreatitis
Budd–Chiari syndrome	Gastritis	
	Myocardial infarction	

Right lumbar	Periumbilical	Left lumbar
Renal calculi	Early appendicitis	Renal calculi
	Gastroenteritis	
	Small bowel obstruction	
	Gallstones	
	Ruptured aortic aneurysm	

Right lower quadrant	Suprapubic	Left lower quadrant
Appendicitis	Urinary tract infection	Diverticulitis
Salpingitis	Uterine fibroids	Salpingitis
Inflammatory bowel disease		Irritable bowel syndrome
Ectopic pregnancy		Inflammatory bowel disease
Inguinal hernia		Inguinal hernia
Mesenteric adenitis		Ectopic pregnancy

overlooked because of other major orthopedic injuries. Progress of the pain will help to differentiate 'constant' pain from 'periodic' pain. Most abdominal pains are intermittent except for pains due to pancreatic carcinoma, dissecting abdominal aneurysm and the referred pains of pneumonia and myocardial infarction. Periodic pains originating from the proximal gut tend to have a diurnal variation, but those from symptomatic gallstones tend to be separated by long periods of remission. Peptic ulcer disease pain can be continuous but of varying severity.

Severity

Severity of the pain is often related to the severity of the underlying disorder. It is always useful to ask the patient to grade the pain on a scale of 1 to 10, where 0 is no pain and 10 being the worst pain imaginable. As an example, the pain of biliary or renal colic or mesenteric infarction is of high intensity compared to the pain of gastroenteritis, which is less marked. However, pain intensity is very subjective and depends on patients' personality and previous experiences of pain. Patients on steroids and elderly patients typically have less pain. Painless perforation of duodenal ulcer in the elderly is not uncommon.

Aggravating and relieving factors

Patients should be asked about aggravating and relieving factors for the pain. When food affects the pain, the source is usually the GI tract. The pain of mesenteric ischemia usually starts within 1 hour of eating while that of a duodenal ulcer is often relieved by eating and recurs when the stomach has emptied. Some body positions influence pain – pain from pancreatitis is relieved by sitting up and leaning forwards. Peritonitis causes patients to lie still as movement worsens pain. Abdominal pain worsened by coughing or sneezing implies that it is arising from the abdominal wall. Patients with irritable bowel syndrome often have lower abdominal pain eased by defecation.

Associated gastrointestinal symptoms

It is very important to explore associated GI symptoms. Weight loss may imply malignancy or malabsorption; nausea and vomiting can be due to intestinal obstruction; diarrhea or constipation with bleeding per rectum is suggestive of colonic pathology.

Physical examination

A complete and thorough examination with emphasis on the abdominal, rectal, and pelvic regions is crucial along with an examination of other relevant systems.

General examination

The general appearance and the level of comfort of the patient should be noted. Patients with biliary or renal colic writhe in agony. Peripheral signs in the form of pallor, jaundice, lymphadenopathy and measurement of vital signs in the form of temperature, blood pressure and pulse rate should be part of the initial assessment. A urinalysis will shed important clues in patients with pain arising from the genitourinary tract and should not be neglected. Fever is significant but its absence, especially in the elderly or immunocompromised patient, does not rule out serious illness.

Abdominal examination

A quick inspection of the abdomen from the viewpoint of the end of the bed can reveal changes in the shape or symmetry of the abdomen. Scars from previous procedures may have some bearing on the cause of the patient's current symptoms. For example, intestinal obstruction is more likely to be secondary to adhesions if there is a history of previous laparotomy.

Always ask about the exact site of abdominal pain and reassure the patient before proceeding to palpate the abdomen. Palpation will help to detect enlarged organs or masses. Muscular rigidity or 'guarding' is an important and early sign of peritoneal inflammation. Unilateral guarding is associated with a focal inflammatory mass, for example, appendicular abscess. Guarding is not seen in deeper sources of pain, for example, renal colic or pancreatitis.

Auscultation of the abdomen for bowel sounds helps to differentiate paralytic ileus, where there is a lack of bowel sounds, from early bowel obstruction where the sounds are abnormally active and high-pitched. Presence of a friction rub over the spleen may signify an infarct while a systolic bruit over the liver is heard in some cases of hepatoma. 'Succussion splash' heard well over 2 hours after food or drink is a feature of gastric outlet obstruction but is rarely heard.

The rectal examination forms an important part of evaluation for all patients with abdominal pain. Fecal impaction, especially in the elderly, is a common cause of abdominal pain while rectal tenderness is typical of retrocecal appendicitis. A pelvic examination should be considered if the history is suggestive of genitourinary pathology. In males, examination of the testes is important, as seminomas are typically painless. Abdominal examination is incomplete without examination of the hernial orifices. Lastly, abdominal wall pathologies such as herpes zoster or abdominal muscle tenderness should be considered.

Investigations

The history and examination usually indicates which investigations will be necessary. A plain radiograph of the abdomen is often useful in patients with acute abdominal pain. A judicious use of a combination of the laboratory tests and radiological investigations should help to identify the cause of abdominal pain (see *Table 6.3*).

Table 6.3. Useful investigations for abdominal pain

Diagnostic tests	
Full blood count, electrolytes, amylase; liver function tests, glucose	Excludes metabolic cause for abdominal pain
Urinalysis; urine for human chorionic gonadotropin	Detects pyuria or hematuria; pregnancy in childbearing age
Electrocardiogram	Ischemic heart disease
Erect chest and abdominal radiography	Bowel perforation or obstruction
Ultrasound of the abdomen and pelvis	Gallstones, hepatic metastases, pelvic organ pathology
Gastroscopy	Peptic ulcer disease, gastritis, gastric cancer
Computed tomography	Pancreatic, appendicular, small and large bowel pathology
Endoscopic retrograde cholangiopancreatography (ERCP)	Pancreatitis, obstructive jaundice
Endoscopic ultrasound (EUS)	Biliary stones, sphincter of Oddi dysfunction
Magnetic resonance cholangiopancreatography (MRCP)	Biliary stones, sphincter of Oddi dysfunction

Common clinical dilemmas

The causes of most cases of abdominal pain become obvious on the standard line of investigations. However, there are certain causes of abdominal pain that can pose great difficulties in diagnosis and/or management to a gastroenterologist, and these are discussed below.

Post-cholecystectomy syndrome

Sphincter of Oddi (SO) dysfunction

The basic abnormality is either a stenosis of the SO or biliary dyskinesia. The clinical presentation is usually a biliary type of pain or recurrent pancreatitis. Sphincter of Oddi dysfunction is most commonly recognized in post-cholecystectomy patients though the actual prevalence of this condition is less than 1% in this group. The 'gold standard' for diagnosis is SO manometry, which is performed during ERCP, however, the test carries a higher risk of pancreatitis, of up to 17%. Various less invasive tests in the form of provocative tests have been evaluated but none has proven to be consistently reliable. The best-studied classification of SO dysfunction is the Milwaukee Biliary Group Classification. This is based on a number of laboratory, clinical and radiological features (see *Table 6.4*).

Table 6.4. Milwaukee Biliary Group Classification of sphincter of Oddi dysfunction

Groups	Clinical features	Treatment options
Type I	Biliary type pain Abnormal aminotransferases more than twice normal Dilated common bile duct > 10 mm Delayed drainage of ERCP contrast after > 45 minutes	Sphincterotomy – 90% successful
Type II	Biliary type pain Any one or more of the other above criteria	Sphincterotomy – < 50% success
Type III	Biliary type pain alone	Controversial; studies awaited

Biliary manometry in type I SO dysfunction demonstrates an increased basal sphincter pressure which fails to relax with smooth muscle relaxants. Manometric studies are generally not needed for this group of patients. However, manometry in types II and III shows a range of abnormalities including sphincter spasm, increased phasic contraction frequency, and paradoxical response to administration of cholecystokinin.

Treatment is aimed at improving the impaired flow of biliary secretions into the duodenum. Pharmacological agents are worth a trial but their benefits are limited by the vasodilating side effects. Calcium channel blockers (nifedipine) and nitrates are the most commonly used. Endoscopic sphincterotomy is beneficial in 90% of patients with type I SO dysfunction, however the benefit is substantially less in patients with types II and III SO dysfunction.

Our practice, for patients with biliary type of pain and dilated common bile duct where no other cause has been found, is to try maximum tolerable doses of nifedipine. Failing this, an ERCP with sphincterotomy is considered. Sphincterotomy should not be undertaken lightly in such patients as it carries a substantial risk of acute pancreatitis (25%) and duodenal perforation (2%). The risks of developing acute pancreatitis can be reduced by the use of a temporary pancreatic stent.

Irritable bowel or biliary dyskinesia

Far more common than sphincter of Oddi dysfunction is the patient who has persistent right upper quadrant pain following a cholecystectomy but all investigations (including LFTs, ultrasound, ERCP and biliary manometry) prove normal. These patients almost certainly represent a variant of irritable bowel and can be difficult to treat. It is our practice to adopt the following management approach:

- Reassure the patient there is no structural abnormality and in particular no gallstones
- Try a fat-free diet
- Antispasmodics: Colofac®, Buscopan®, Colpermin®
- Calcium channel blocker
- Motival® 10 mg three times daily often helpful in resistant cases

Chronic pancreatitis

The management of pain in chronic pancreatitis can be difficult. Pain is the most common symptom that brings the patient to medical attention, and can range from mild and intermittent, to constant and disabling. Patients should be advised to abstain from alcohol. Small meals, low in fat, may also be helpful.

First-line therapy should always be with basic analgesics like acetominaphen (paracetamol), dihydrocodeine, NSAIDs, etc. More often, narcotic analgesics are required to control pain. As narcotic dependence can become an important problem, a single practitioner should be identified as the designated prescriber. Before considering long-term narcotic analgesics, short-term hospitalization with the patient kept 'nil by mouth' to minimize pancreatic stimulation and simultaneous brief course of narcotics with low-dose amitriptyline and NSAIDs may break the pain cycle.

Pancreatic enzyme supplements seem to benefit patients with mild to moderate disease but the results of studies are variable because of a high placebo response rate (33%). The rationale for this therapy is based on the fact that oral administration of trypsin will suppress the feedback loop in the duodenum which regulates the release of cholecystokinin (CCK), the hormone which stimulates the exocrine pancreas.

The use of octreotide in chronic pancreatitis pain is still experimental but preliminary reports have shown promise. Patients with intractable pain in spite of aggressive noninvasive treatment should undergo CT of the pancreas to look for complications (e.g. pseudocysts) and ERCP to assess the pancreatic and biliary tree. Stones in the pancreatic duct can be removed and strictures of the pancreatic duct may be considered for stenting. The studies on the use of plastic endoprostheses across strictures in the pancreatic duct were largely uncontrolled, but symptoms improved in a selected group of patients (50%).

Surgical drainage operations like pancreaticojejunostomy can successfully decompress pancreatic ducts which are larger than 8 mm. In patients with nondilated pancreatic ducts, the disease is largely parenchymal and partial or total pancreatectomy may be considered if symptoms are intractable. Celiac plexus block with alcohol or steroids is useful for unremitting pain.

Irritable bowel syndrome (see also Chapter 12)

Occasionally patients with irritable bowel have quite severe, chronic pain which is difficult to treat. Probably the most important component of treatment is establishing a strong physician–patient relationship. It is very useful to discuss with the patient the chronic and benign nature of this disease, that the diagnosis is not likely to be changed and that there is no change in life expectancy.

Dietary modifications in the form of avoidance of foods that increase flatulence (onions, beans, celery, apricots, Brussels sprouts, bananas) and increased intake of fiber is a good starting point. A careful dietary history will help to identify the offending foods. Up to 50% of patients respond to an exclusion diet. A small number of patients, particularly those whose symptoms started following a bout of gastroenteritis or oral antibiotics, respond to the Brostoff diet (see Further reading). This diet separates protein and carbohydrate and is said to reduce gut fermentation.

Pharmacological agents are only adjuncts to the treatment of irritable bowel syndrome. Antispasmodic agents are beneficial in patients with postprandial abdominal pain and bloatedness. Antidepressants have analgesic properties independent on their mood improving effects and are helpful for pain in irritable bowel syndrome. The possible mechanism is through release of endogenous endorphins. The dose of tricyclic antidepressants required for abdominal pain is much lower than that required for treatment of depression. The newer selective serotonin re-uptake inhibitors (SSRI) are probably as useful as tricyclic antidepressants and less sedating. Hypnosis, biofeedback and psychotherapy help to reduce anxiety, increase patient awareness and responsibility and improve pain tolerance. These are particularly useful for motivated patients with complex psychosocial factors.

Patients with intractable pain despite the above measures should be referred to the pain clinic.

Chronic mesenteric ischemia

Patients with chronic mesenteric ischemia present with 'intestinal angina' which is characterized by recurrent acute episodes of abdominal pain during times of heightened intestinal demand (postprandial). The typical patient has arterial disease with underlying atherosclerotic vascular disease and a significant history of smoking.

The 'gold standard' test for mesenteric ischemia is angiography. In experienced hands, duplex ultrasound can visualize 80–90% of celiac and superior mesenteric artery stenosis and therefore is an important screening tool prior to invasive tests.

Treatment options are:

Box 6.2	Clinical features of chronic mesenteric ischemia
	• Postprandial pain which starts within the first hour after eating and lasts for up to 4 hours • Pain usually dull and aching • Loss of weight, often more than 10% of the body weight • Diarrhea due to malabsorption

- Percutaneous transluminal angioplasty with or without stent – these are preferred to surgical reconstruction in patients who are poor surgical candidates
- Surgical revascularization with reconstruction of the splanchnic arteries is a relatively safe procedure with morbidity and mortality between 2% and 5%
- Octreotide has been successfully used for pain relief in patients with mesenteric ischemia who are unsuitable for any major intervention

Chronic abdominal pain due to intra-abdominal malignancy

Pain due to intra-abdominal malignancy is typically visceral in nature and therefore poorly localized. This is often accompanied by nausea and vomiting. This can be referred to various places: for example, retroperitoneal tumors cause back pain; diaphragmatic irritation from hepatic capsular involvement causes right shoulder pain. The pain of pancreatic cancer is particularly severe and may be amenable to celiac plexus blockade.

Box 6.3	Typical features of abdominal wall pain
	• Pain intensity related to posture • Pain not related to food or bowel action • Pain often constant and fluctuating; rarely episodic • Abdominal tenderness unchanged or increased when abdominal wall is tensed (Carnett's sign) • Presence of trigger points along the lateral margins of the rectus abdominis muscles • Absence of features of intra-abdominal pathology like nausea, vomiting, pain related to food or bowel action, weight loss, bowel irregularity, anemia and abnormal blood results

A detailed description and approach for pain relief in patients with terminal disease is found in Chapter 22.

Chronic abdominal wall pain

The abdominal wall as source of pain is often overlooked and this can result in prolonged, expensive and unnecessary investigations. In most cases, the diagnosis can be made after a detailed history and physical examination. Radiological investigations such as ultrasound or CT scan should be requested with a specific clinical diagnosis in mind. Either CT or MRI studies of the spine may be helpful for spinal nerve irritation.

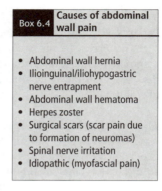

Box 6.4 Causes of abdominal wall pain

- Abdominal wall hernia
- Ilioinguinal/iliohypogastric nerve entrapment
- Abdominal wall hematoma
- Herpes zoster
- Surgical scars (scar pain due to formation of neuromas)
- Spinal nerve irritation
- Idiopathic (myofascial pain)

The most important management step is to reassure the patient. Undertaking unnecessary investigations when this diagnosis is evident would only reinforce the patient's anxiety. A trial of injection of the most tender spot (trigger point) with a local anesthetic both helps to treat as well as confirm the abdominal wall as the pain source. Traditionally a few tenths of milliliters of 1% lidocaine (lignocaine) is injected into the most tender spot. For more permanent relief, a mixture of local anesthetic and corticosteroid is used. In some patients, the presence of depression or other psychological dysfunction causes the pain to seem out of proportion to other findings; such patients benefit from antidepressant therapy.

Persistent pain in spite of the above measures should be referred to the specialist pain management team.

Further reading

Brostoff, J. and Gamlin, L. (1998) *The Complete Guide to Food Allergy and Intolerance.* Bloomsbury.

Wall, P.D. and Melzack, R. (1999) Chapter 32. In: *Textbook of Pain*, 4th Edn. Churchill Livingstone.

7 Abnormal Liver Function Tests

Hyder Hussaini

Introduction

This chapter will focus on the management of patients who present with abnormal liver function tests (LFTs) or established cirrhosis, and the investigations required for the new outpatient, including the role of liver biopsy.

Patients presenting with abnormal liver function tests

Serum alanine aminotransferase (ALT), aspartate aminotransferase (AST), collectively termed transaminases, alkaline phosphatase (ALP) or gamma-glutamyltransferase (GGT) are commonly referred to as LFTs, although they are essentially markers of hepatobiliary disease. In contrast, serum albumin and prothrombin time reflect actual liver synthetic function.

Although 1–6% of asymptomatic individuals will have abnormal LFTs, the prevalence of liver disease in the general population is estimated to be only 2–3%. Thus, abnormal LFTs in an asymptomatic patient are poorly predictive of any serious liver pathology, but may be due to significant treatable liver disease. A crude guide to the etiology of abnormal LFTs may be derived from the pattern of transaminase or ALP rise.

Clinical assessment (see also Chapter 3)

Marked elevation of transaminase (> 300 IU/l) or ALP (> 2 × upper limit of normal) should prompt immediate further investigation and clinical assessment. In contrast, it is our practice only to further investigate patients with mild or moderate abnormal transaminase that persists for more than 6 months. Since transaminase levels can fluctuate in diseases such as chronic hepatitis C, it is the chronicity of transaminase abnormality rather than the magnitude of elevation that is probably most relevant.

Prior to outpatients, all patients have a full screen for etiological causes of chronic liver disease (see *Table 7.1*). Abdominal ultrasound is performed in all patients prior to the outpatient visit, in particular to examine for obstructive biliary disease, focal hepatic abnormalities and hepatic infiltration. In clinic, particular reference is made to symptoms of chronic liver disease, alcohol intake, recent medication, risk factors for viral hepatitis acquisition, body weight and signs of chronic liver disease. Cholestatic features (pruritus and raised ALP) may occur in primary biliary cirrhosis (PBC) or be associated with drug treatment.

Table 7.1. Noninvasive investigations to 'screen' for the cause of underlying liver disease

	Screening test	Further investigations
Hepatitis B (HBV)	HB s Antigen	HB e Antigen/antibody HBV DNA
Hepatitis C (HCV)	HCV ELISA antibody	HCV RNA
Primary biliary cirrhosis	Immunoglobulins (raised IgM) Antimitochondrial antibodies	M2 antibody
Autoimmune hepatitis	Immunoglobulins (raised IgG) Smooth muscle antibodies Anti nuclear antibodies LKM antibodies Antimitochondrial antibodies	
Genetic hemochromatosis	Raised transferrin saturation Ferritin raised	HFE gene analysis
Alpha-1-antitrypsin deficiency	Low alpha-1-antitrypsin	Genotype studies
Wilson's disease	Low ceruloplasmin Raised 24-h urinary copper excretion	Penicillamine challenge
Primary sclerosing cholangitis	Antineutrophil antibody positive	Cholangiography

Predominant elevation of alkaline phosphatase

ALP can be elevated due to cholestatic liver disease, such as PBC, primary sclerosing cholangitis (PSC) or obstruction of the biliary tree. Raised IgM and antimitochondrial antibodies with M2 antibody are specific for PBC. Anticytoplasmic antibody titers (ANCA) are positive in 65–85% of PSC patients. Bone disease in the elderly, such as Paget's disease, can cause marked elevation of ALP, although isoenzyme analysis distinguishes the source of ALP. Alternatively, GGT can be used as a surrogate marker, because in the presence of elevated GGT, elevated ALP is likely to be hepatic in origin. A modest isolated rise in the elderly patient ($< 2 \times$ the upper limit of normal) is generally of less concern than in younger patients. In patients with elevated ALP of hepatic origin, abdominal ultrasound is essential to exclude biliary obstruction secondary to 'silent' gallstone disease, infiltration of the liver with metastatic disease or liver abscess, leading to a predominant rise in ALP.

Predominant raised transaminase

The degree of elevation of transaminase, and whether or not this is a persistent, solitary abnormality in LFTs or fluctuating elevation, is of some help in elucidating a diagnosis. The degree of elevation in transaminase covers a continuum of hepatological disease from steatohepatitis to acute viral hepatitis. Severe elevation of transaminase (> 1000 IU/l) occurs in acute viral hepatitis, acute ischemic hepatitis (usually seen in hospital patients) and after paracetamol overdose. However, it is the asymptomatic patient with a mild or moderate rise in transaminase that causes concern.

A mild rise in transaminase (less than a two- to threefold rise over normal) is often due to steatohepatitis (either nonalcoholic or alcohol induced) or concurrent drug therapy. Chronic viral hepatitis, due to either hepatitis B or C, may lead to mild or moderate (2–5 × upper limit of normal) rise in transaminase. Alcohol-induced liver disease, autoimmune-induced liver disease, genetic hemochromatosis, and alpha-one antitrypsin deficiency can also lead to mild or moderate transaminase elevations.

Aspartate transaminase/alanine transaminase ratio

An AST/ALT ratio greater than 2.0 is highly suggestive of alcoholic liver disease. A ratio less than 1.0 can occur in nonalcoholic liver disease patients who develop cirrhosis, although it is also a good marker of chronic viral hepatitis. Practically, there are now better investigations to discriminate between these disorders and, more pragmatically, many biochemistry departments will only measure ALT, thus AST/ALT ratios are seldom used in clinical practice.

Management

If the noninvasive screening investigations outlined above are nondiagnostic and LFT abnormalities persist, then liver biopsy may be required. In general, if transaminase elevation is less than 2–3 × the upper limit of normal, patients are advised to lose weight if obese and, in those that drink alcohol, to abstain for 3 months. Patients with persistent elevation of transaminase or the younger patient with an isolated rise in hepatic ALP (rarer) may require liver biopsy and should be fully counseled with regard to this procedure.

Cirrhosis

Asymptomatic patients with cirrhosis may present with abnormal laboratory investigations (elevated serum aminotransferases, hypoalbuminemia, prolonged prothrombin time, thrombocytopenia) or unexpected clinical findings of stigmata of chronic liver disease, hepatomegaly or splenomegaly. Alternatively, patients may need follow-up after hospital admission following complications of cirrhosis, such as ascites or variceal bleeding.

Etiology

Alcohol-related liver disease and chronic hepatitis C are probably the commonest causes for cirrhosis in the UK. Clinical history can give clues to specific diagnoses; alcohol history and risk factors for hepatitis should be sought. A history of fatigue, pruritus, skin hyperpigmentation and xanthelasma may suggest a diagnosis of PBC. PSC and autoimmune hepatitis are associated with inflammatory bowel disease. A familial history of liver disease can be associated with genetic hemochromatosis and alpha-1 antitrypsin deficiency.

Initial management

Measurement of serum albumin, bilirubin and prothrombin time are the most useful guides to hepatic function, which, in combination with clinical features of encephalopathy and ascites, can give long-term prognostic information using the Child–Pugh classification (see *Table 7.2*). Patients with Child's B and C disease should be considered for liver transplant assessment, if appropriate. A predominant rise in serum ALP may suggest a diagnosis of PBC. Serum transaminase is seldom of any use in helping with diagnosis of the cause of cirrhosis and is often normal. Abdominal ultrasound to assess the portal vein patency and examination of the liver for focal abnormalities such as hepatoma, together with measurement of alpha-fetoprotein (AFP) is essential. AFP is often elevated in cirrhosis. However, a serial rise in AFP or values greater than 100 IU/l should prompt further investigation such as CT, hepatic angiography or magnetic resonance imaging (MRI) of the liver. A full 'liver screen' (see *Table 7.1*) can be performed prior to the outpatient visit. If possible, the underlying cause should be treated. Liver biopsy, in some but not all patients, may be required to confirm the diagnosis of cirrhosis (see section on Liver biopsy).

Table 7.2. Child–Pugh classification

Parameter	1	2	3
Ascites	None	Moderate	Severe
Encephalopathy	None	Grade 1–2	Grade 3–4
Albumin (g/l)	> 35	28–35	< 28
Bilirubin (mmol/l)	< 32	32–55	> 55
Prothrombin time (seconds > control)	1–3	4–6	> 6
(INR)	1.7	1.8–2.3	> 2.3

Child–Pugh score:
< 6:   Grade A, well-compensated chronic liver disease (1- and 2-year survival 100% and 85%, respectively).
7–9:   Grade B, moderate compensated chronic liver disease (1- and 2-year survival 80% and 60%, respectively).
> 10: Grade C, poorly compensated chronic liver disease (1- and 2-year survival 45% and 35%, respectively).

Outpatient follow-up for complications of cirrhosis

In most cirrhotic patients or those with advanced fibrosis screening for varices, hepatic osteodystrophy and hepatocellular carcinoma should be performed.

Approximately 60% of patients with cirrhosis will have upper GI varices. As treatment with propranolol or nadolol is an effective primary prophylaxis, all patients with cirrhosis should undergo upper GI endoscopy. Patients with large esophageal varices at endoscopy should enter a banding program as primary prophylaxis.

Both osteomalacia and osteoporosis are common (30–40% of patients) and occur in patients with cholestatic and noncholestatic chronic liver disease. Osteomalacia in patients with liver disease occurs particularly with cholestatic disease, such as PBC secondary to vitamin D deficiency, and responds to administration of vitamin D. In patients with cholestatic liver disease, serum calcium, phosphate and vitamin D are measured at diagnosis and every 3 years. Patients with vitamin D deficiency should start vitamin D supplements, initially vitamin D (400–800 IU/day), together with calcium (1 g/day). Serum vitamin D is re-checked 3 months later and, if not within normal limits, 1-alpha-calcidol (20 µg/day) can then be used.

Patients with cirrhosis or chronic cholestatic disorders (bilirubin > 50 µmol/l for more than 6 months), such as PBC, are at particular risk of osteoporosis. Risk factors for osteoporosis in any patient with liver disease include prolonged steroid administration (e.g. patients with autoimmune liver disease or after liver transplantation), and those with hypogonadism, family history of early maternal hip fracture and low body mass index (BMI < 19 kg/m^2). These patients undergo bone densitometry, as there is an increased risk of spontaneous bone fracture. We use dual emission X-ray densitometry (DEXA) to assess the risk for bone fracture. Lumbar spine and femoral neck bone mineral density (BMD) is calculated (g/cm^2) and Z scores subsequently derived, corrected for age and sex. The Z score for BMD is the number of standard deviations above or below the mean BMD for an age- and sex-matched normal population. Patients with osteopenia (Z score < −1.5) are treated with calcium supplementation with repeat densitometry every 2–3 years. All female patients eligible for hormone replacement therapy (HRT) treatment are advised to start HRT. Patients with osteoporosis (Z score < −2.5) should undergo further investigations, including thyroid function test, bone function tests (25-OH vitamin D and parathyroid hormone (PTH) if persistent hypocalcemia), serum estradiol follicular stimulating hormone and luteinizing hormone in females, and testosterone and sex hormone-binding globulin in males [expressed as a ratio (< 0.3 = hypogonadism) or free testosterone]. Hypogonadal patients are treated with replacement therapy. Those patients intolerant of replacement therapy or who are eugonadal receive bisphosphonate therapy. We then perform annual densitometry to assess any disease progression. Any patients with liver disease and spontaneous bone fracture do not require densitometry, but appropriate treatment with HRT (if hypogonadism is present) or bisphosphonates.

The incidence of hepatocellular carcinoma in patients with cirrhosis is approximately 1–6% per year, with particular risk for patients with cirrhosis due to hepatitis B and C or genetic hemochromatosis. We currently check AFP, and offer ultrasound every 6 months in those patients with cirrhosis who are fit enough to be surgical candidates for transplantation or hepatectomy, should a tumor be discovered. This remains controversial and is not proven on a cost-effective basis (see also Chapter 10, section on Screening for hepatocellular carcinoma).

Liver biopsy

All biopsies within our unit are ultrasound guided. In patients who are at low risk of bleeding, the biopsy is performed as a day case. These patients will have someone who can stay with them overnight. High-risk patients (*Box 7.1*) have liver biopsy performed with overnight stay, with the biopsy performed either via the transjugular route or as a 'plugged' biopsy. We will normally administer fresh frozen plasma (4 units) for percutaneous biopsy if the international normalised rate (INR) is between 1.4 and 2.0, with 20 mg vitamin K given intravenously 24 h beforehand. If the INR is greater than 2.0 or platelet count less than 50 000, then biopsy is performed by the transjugular route.

The nature, indications, alternatives and relative risks of liver biopsy, including hemorrhage (one in 200–300), perforated viscus (one in 1000) and death (between one in 1000 and one in 10 000) are discussed with all patients. We tell patients that postprocedural discomfort occurs in one in three patients, although severe pain can occur (1–3%).

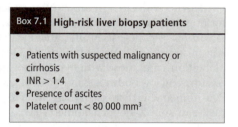

Box 7.1 **High-risk liver biopsy patients**

- Patients with suspected malignancy or cirrhosis
- INR > 1.4
- Presence of ascites
- Platelet count < 80 000 mm^3

In patients with early PBC and positive M2 antibodies, liver biopsy may be normal and thus is not performed. Similarly, patients with genetic hemochromatosis (on HFE gene mutation analysis) and normal LFTs, with a ferritin less than 1000 µg/l, are unlikely to have cirrhosis; thus, biopsy is not indicated to manage their condition further. The diagnosis of PSC is radiological (ERCP or MRCP) rather than histological; thus, we do not consider this an indication for liver biopsy. We perform liver biopsy in most patients with nonalcoholic steatohepatitis specifically to look for features suggestive of progressive disease such as fibrosis, especially in those over the age of 45 with obesity or diabetes, since fibrosis is more likely. In patients with suspected cirrhosis or chronic hepatitis, we will perform liver biopsy to confirm the diagnosis and assist in prognostic assessment. However, in noncompliant patients with alcohol dependency and those with severe comorbid disease, biopsy is not performed, as we do not feel that management is affected. The decision to biopsy 'high-risk' patients needs to be balanced with the potential benefits in each individual case.

Summary

Many patients with abnormal LFTs will not have serious liver pathology. The decision to investigate further is often made based on chronicity of LFT abnormalities and, to a degree, the magnitude of these abnormalities. Preclinic virology, biochemistry and immunology, together with ultrasound, can assist on a one-stop approach in clinic (see also Chapter 3). These investigations, together with careful history and examination will often elucidate the diagnosis. In patients with compensated cirrhosis, prevention of variceal hemorrhage, treatment of hepatic osteodystrophy and screening for hepatoma are key management issues in addition to treatment of the underlying cause of cirrhosis. Although liver biopsy has a role in assessing prognosis, it is rarely required to confirm the diagnosis alone because of noninvasive hepatic investigations.

Further reading

Collier, J.D., Ninkovic, M. and Compston, J.E. (2002) Guidelines on the management of osteoporosis associated with chronic liver disease. *Gut* **50** (Suppl. 1): i1–i9.

Grant, A. and Neuberger, J. (1999) Guidelines on the use of liver biopsy in clinical practice. British Society of Gastroenterology.

8 | Change in Bowel Habit: Constipation/Unexplained Diarrhea

Joy Worthington and John Wong

Introduction

Constipation and diarrhea are common presenting complaints in the GI outpatient clinic. The aim of this chapter is to provide a diagnostic and management approach for these symptoms, rather than an exhaustive list of differential diagnoses. Diarrhea is defined as the passage of greater than three loose stools or stool output of greater than 200 g in 24 h. Acute diarrhea is often dealt with in primary care. In the majority of cases, it will be self-limiting but in others, it runs a more chronic course. Patients with chronic diarrhea, as defined by diarrhea lasting longer than 3 weeks, will often require additional investigation in the secondary care setting.

Normal bowel frequency ranges from three times a day to three times a week. The definition of constipation consists of a combination of decreased bowel frequency (less than three times a week), straining, hard stools or incomplete evacuation more than 25% of the time.

A change in bowel habit is an important feature in the history and requires further investigation. The main focus of assessment is to differentiate between functional and organic causes for the symptoms. New-onset diarrhea is one of the major criteria for urgent referral under the 2-week standard according to Department of Health (DoH) guidelines (*Box 8.1*).

Colorectal carcinoma is the foremost concern for the patient or the GPs. When seeing a new patient with a change in bowel habit, it helps to understand the background of the referrals.

Some GPs nowadays initiate some form of investigations before making the referral. These may have been unremarkable or showed incidental abnormality that may be irrelevant. A working diagnosis (such as irritable bowel syndrome; IBS) may have been made but patients remain symptomatic despite empirical treatment. Some patients wish a second (specialist) opinion and often require reassurance rather than another repeated exhaustive list of screening

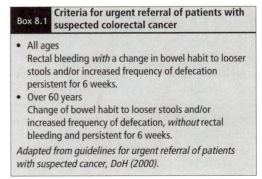

Box 8.1	Criteria for urgent referral of patients with suspected colorectal cancer

- All ages
  Rectal bleeding *with* a change in bowel habit to looser stools and/or increased frequency of defecation persistent for 6 weeks.
- Over 60 years
  Change of bowel habit to looser stools and/or increased frequency of defecation, *without* rectal bleeding and persistent for 6 weeks.

Adapted from guidelines for urgent referral of patients with suspected cancer, DoH (2000).

tests to exacerbate their anxiety. In other patients, the results may be equivocal and/or diagnosis remains uncertain, making further tests justified. Some patients are found to have definite pathology such as colonic polyp. These patients require specific advice and a formulated plan of management.

An approach to a patient with chronic diarrhea

History

Meaning of diarrhea

Find out whether this consists of an increase in bowel frequency, loose stool or both. A stool description of steatorrhea provides a clue towards fat malabsorption.

Duration of symptoms

Establish whether the onset of diarrhea is acute or gradual. Acute diarrhea suggests an infective etiology, whereas a long history without sinister features is more indicative of a functional problem. The pattern of diarrhea is also important. Intermittent diarrhea alternating with constipation, often in the morning and with mucus, is suggestive of IBS. Nocturnal diarrhea suggests an organic cause.

Preceding/precipitating events

Any history of traveling to an exotic part of the world or other affected family members would suggest an infective cause. Patients may recollect ingestion of contaminated foodstuffs to suggest food poisoning. A memorable episode of gastroenteritis prior to symptom onset points towards post infective IBS or transient lactose intolerance. A significant change of diet, for example a weight-reducing diet, may be relevant.

Associated features

Abdominal pain with diarrhea is a helpful diagnostic feature. The differential diagnosis includes IBS, inflammatory bowel disease (IBD) and ischemic colitis. Young patients with pain associated with a change in stool frequency or consistency, and relieved by defecation, are typical of IBS (see Chapter 12). These patients often have symptoms that worsen with periods of stress and anxiety. The pain associated with ischemic colitis is often related to meals and patients can have associated weight loss. The severity can vary, vomiting is often a feature and the diarrhea can be bloody. Patients are usually elderly and have a history of atherosclerosis.

Bloody diarrhea also offers diagnostic clues suggestive of an organic cause (see *Box 8.2*).

Associated weight loss is a worrying feature and, if substantial, may be suggestive of an underlying malignancy or secondary to malabsorption. Anorexia and anemia both suggest an organic cause.

Past medical/surgical history

Past medical history, including history of radiotherapy, previous surgery, history of eating disorders, hyperthyroidism, diabetes mellitus and Addison's disease, may suggest an organic cause for the diarrheal symptoms. For instance, patients with right hemicolectomy/terminal ileal resection are prone to bile salt malabsorption or bacterial overgrowth.

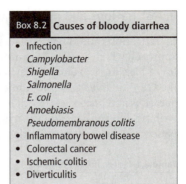

Box 8.2	**Causes of bloody diarrhea**

- Infection
  Campylobacter
  Shigella
  Salmonella
  E. coli
  Amoebiasis
  Pseudomembranous colitis
- Inflammatory bowel disease
- Colorectal cancer
- Ischemic colitis
- Diverticulitis

Sexual history may be important, as infections causing diarrhea or proctitis can occur without immunodeficiency in homosexual men. An acute diarrheal illness can also be a presentation of acquired immune deficiency syndrome (AIDS) as either infective diarrhea or as human immunodeficiency virus (HIV) enteropathy. No causative agent is found in HIV enteropathy and a partial villous atrophy occurs.

Family history

A family history of inflammatory bowel disease, colon cancer or celiac disease with symptoms suggestive of any of these is of relevance to calculating the risk of the patient having the same disease, leading to a lower threshold for endoscopic investigations.

Drug history

Take a full drug history looking for the use of magnesium-containing antacids; PPIs, antibiotics; antidepressants (SSRI) which can all cause diarrhea. Remember surreptitious laxative use as a potential cause for diarrhea.

Examination

A thorough systematic examination is necessary. Physical signs may offer vital clues to the diagnosis and guidance for the most appropriate investigation.

Examine the patient for any signs of anemia, clubbing, lymphadenopathy or goiter. Clubbing can be seen in IBD especially Crohn's disease (CD). Erythema nodosum and pyoderma gangrenosum are extraintestinal features of IBD. Dermatitis herpetiformis is an itchy vesicular rash found mainly on the elbows and buttocks of 2% of those with celiac disease.

Examine the abdomen for any masses or hepatosplenomegaly. A right iliac fossa mass may be an inflammatory mass of CD in a younger patient or a cecal tumor in an older patient. Surgical scars should be noted. A rectal examination is essential to look for tumors or impaction of feces.

Investigations and management

Investigation should be directed at the most likely diagnosis. We suggest a staged approach which reserves the more uncommon tests for 'unexplained' diarrhea. A list of baseline 'screening' investigations may be helpful if not already initiated by the GP (see *Table 8.1*). Stool microscopy should be done looking for ova, cysts, parasites and bacteria – in other words, an infective cause of diarrhea. Consider looking for *Clostridium difficile* toxin in debilitated, immunocompromised patients or following antibiotic treatment.

Table 8.1. 'Screening' investigations

	Tests	Rationale
Stool	Microscopy and culture Consider testing for fat globules	Rule out parasitic infection Look for fat malabsorption
Blood tests	U&E, thyroid function, glucose, albumin, CRP, ESR, endomysial antibody immunoglobulins	Detect diabetes mellitus, hyperthyroidism, IBD, celiac disease
	Consider testing for folate, serum B_{12}, Ca^{2+}, Mg^{2+} and Zn^{2+}	Malabsorption syndrome

U&E, urea and electrolytes; CRP, C-reactive protein: ESR, erynrocyte sedimentation rate; IBD, inflammatory bowel disease.

General management points

The treatment of diarrhea obviously depends on the cause. Any offending drugs that may be contributory to diarrhea can be stopped short term. Diarrhea due to specific diagnoses such as hyperthyroidism should improve with treatment of the underlying problem. Rehydration is an important general measure. Infants and the elderly are at considerable risk if not adequately rehydrated. A postural drop in blood pressure or tachycardia suggests severe dehydration, and inpatient treatment with intravenous fluids will be required. Parenteral nutrition may be required in more severe prolonged cases. Empirical treatment with an antibiotic (e.g. ciprofloxacin) may be tried if there is high suspicion of bacterial infection within a community or in a specific patient. However, delaying treatment until confirmation of an infectious cause for the diarrhea is preferable.

Symptomatic treatment for undiagnosed or unexplained diarrhea includes opiate-based drugs, for example codeine phosphate or loperamide. These should not be used in a patient with acute severe colitis. They are otherwise safe agents for symptomatic control, even in infectious diarrhea.

Pending on the results of the screening tests, further investigations can be specifically directed to confirm or refute a working diagnosis (see *Table 8.2*).

A microcytic anemia is commonly due to iron deficiency. This can be confirmed by iron studies showing a low ferritin and iron saturation. Iron deficiency may represent IBD, celiac disease or colon carcinoma. Macrocytosis, often

Table 8.2. Some common working diagnosis of chronic diarrhea

	Working diagnosis	Tests	Management options
Typical history, normal tests and physical examinations	IBS	Avoid unnecessary additional tests	See Chapter 12
Anemia, over the age of 40 with or without sinister symptoms	Colorectal cancer, celiac disease – rule out other sources of blood loss	OGD and D2 biopsy plus colonoscopy	See Chapter 4
Raised inflammatory markers	IBD	Flexible sigmoidoscopy or colonoscopy, small bowel barium studies, ultrasound or CT abdomen if mass identified	See Chapter 11
Strong family history +/− positive endomysial antibody	Celiac disease	OGD and D2 biopsy	See Chapter 15
Increased fat globules in stool	Steatorrhea/ malabsorption syndrome		
	Bacterial overgrowth		Empirical antibiotics
	Pancreatic insufficiency	Tests to identify cause of pancreatic insufficiency, e.g. abdominal X-ray and ultrasound or CT scan for chronic pancreatitis	Pancreatic enzyme supplements
Unremarkable tests and physical examinations	Microscopic colitis – lymphocytic or collagenous colitis	Flexible sigmoidoscopy and random biopsies, also identify melanosis coli	5-ASA agents, consider steroids
	Carbohydrate intolerance Bile salt malabsorption		Empirical dietary exclusion Empirical cholestyramine or Colestipol

IBS, irritable bowel syndrome; EGD, esophagogastroduodenoscopy; IBD, inflammatory bowel disease; CT, computed tomography; 5-ASA agents, aminosalicylate acid.

due to either folate or B_{12} deficiency, may be indicative of celiac disease or terminal ileal CD. Chronic alcohol abuse can also cause macrocytosis and contribute to diarrhea symptoms.

High plasma viscosity and CRP levels may be found in active IBD, infections and carcinoma. However, normal results can occur in both IBD and carcinoma. Low albumin suggests malnourishment. This may be present in inflammatory conditions, malabsorption and carcinoma. Immunoglobulins are low in hypogammaglobulinemia, which can cause villous atrophy and bacterial overgrowth. Serological tests for antibodies to gliadin, endomysium and tissue transglutaminase can be used for screening those with diarrhea for celiac disease.

Table 8.3. Investigations for more difficult cases of chronic diarrhea

Presumed problem	Tests	Brief description	Positive results
Steatorrhea	Fecal fat estimation	3-day stool collection; diet containing 100 g fat per day	> 7 g day^{-1}
	^{14}Carbon triolein breath test	Exhaled $^{14}CO_2$ is measured after ingestion of radiolabelled triolein	Low levels are found in fat malabsorption
Laxative abuse	Urine laxative screen (anthraquinone)	Random urine sample	Positive anthracene test
	Alkalization of stool (phenolphthalein)	Random stool sample	
Lactase deficiency	Lactose tolerance test	50 g oral lactose; blood samples at baseline and intervals	A rise of blood glucose < 20 mg per 100 ml or 1.1 mmol/l above baseline
	Hydrogen breath test	50 g oral lactose; breath measurement every 30–60 min for 2–4 h	> 20 ppm above baseline or clinical symptoms of colic, bloating and/or diarrhea
Pancreatic insufficiency	Pancreolauryl test (aryl esterase)	Two parts: oral esterified and nonesterified fluorescein on 2 separate days; urine collection 10 h each	Normal excretion index > 30%
	NBT-PABA (chymotrypsin)	Oral labelled ^{14}C and free PABA; urine collection for 6 h	Normal excretion index > 50%
	Fecal chymotrypsin	Random stool sample; ELISA test	< 6 U g^{-1} stool
	Fecal elastase 1	Random stool sample; ELISA test	< 200 mg g^{-1} stool
Bacterial overgrowth	^{14}C Glycocholic breath test	Test for bile acid deconjugation	
	^{14}C Xylose breath test	Oral ^{14}C D-xylose with unlabeled D-xylose; measurement of breath $^{14}CO_2$ at intervals	High level of $^{14}CO_2$
Bile salt malabsorption	^{75}SeHCAT	Oral gelatine capsule carrying ^{75}SeHCAT	< 5% retention at day 7
		Measurement of retention at day 0 and day 7	5–10% retention at day 7, possible malabsorption or rapid GI transit
Neuroendocrine malignancy	Fasting gut hormones	Blood sample require rapid processing; for fasting gastrin, discontinue PPI for at least 2 weeks	Abnormal levels require follow up radiological imaging, angiography and venous sampling
Carcinoid syndrome	HIAA	24-h urine collection; dietary restriction	> 7 mg or 37 mmol in 24 h

NBT-PABA, N-benzoyl-L-tyrosyl; PABA, para-amino benzoic acid; ELISA, enzyme-linked immunosorbent assay; PPI, proton pump inhibitor; HIAA, 5-hydroxy-indoleacetic acid.

More specialized investigations may be necessary for those whose diagnosis remains unclear and who remain symptomatic with or without empirical treatment (see *Table 8.3*).

Unexplained diarrhea

If there are no sinister features and the symptoms are controlled with anti-diarrheal agents, no further investigations are necessary. In difficult symptomatic patients with unexplained diarrhea, a brief period of inpatient assessment may be helpful. This can be arranged via a short-stay investigation unit. There are several advantages to this approach. The patient will be under direct nursing observation. Any diarrhea episodes are recorded in a stool chart. The stool can be observed for steatorrhea. Stool and urine sample can be obtained for surreptitious laxative use. Three-day fecal fat collections are rarely performed nowadays (very unpopular with the biochemist!). The patient can be fasted for 24 h whilst maintained on intravenous fluids. The continuation of diarrhea symptoms whilst fasting suggests a secretory cause such as a neuroendocrine tumor. Any patients exhibiting psychiatric symptoms will require a full psychological evaluation.

Malabsorption

This can be broadly subdivided into three types:

- Unabsorbed solutes: poor absorption of sorbitol and fructose cause diarrhea by an osmotic mechanism. This may be a problem when there is excessive consumption of fruits containing these sugars, such as pears, prunes, apples and peaches. These sugars are also used as sweeteners in soft drinks and dieting food.
- Mucosa damage: celiac disease is characterized by villous atrophy, which results in malabsorption of various nutrients. The diagnosis and management for this is discussed in Chapter 15. Certain drugs such as neomycin and colchicine may also cause mucosa damage leading to steatorrhea.
- Maldigestion: pancreatic insufficiency causes maldigestion of carbohydrate, protein and fat, which leads to diarrhea and steatorrhea.

Malabsorption can be associated with weight loss and specific features contributable to the malabsorbed nutrient.

Malabsorption of carbohydrate leads to watery diarrhea with bloating and borborygmi. These general symptoms may be wrongly thought to be secondary to IBS. Note, however, that malabsorption can occur without diarrhea. Weight loss can occur whatever the malabsorption, but protein malabsorption produces visible weight loss and muscle wasting, as well as peripheral edema.

Specific vitamin or mineral deficiencies can cause specific clinical symptoms and signs. For example, calcium and vitamin D deficiency can lead to osteomalacia and osteoporosis.

Investigation of malabsorption

Although endoscopy and biopsy of the second part of the duodenum is often used to diagnose celiac disease, other causes of small bowel malabsorption need to be borne in mind. These include Whipple's disease, CD, lymphoma, giardiasis, hypogammaglobulinemia and amyloidosis.

Jejunal biopsies at enteroscopy can give more information if duodenal biopsies are unhelpful. An aspirate of small intestinal contents can be sent for analysis of *Giardia* infection or aerobic/anaerobic quantitative bacterial culture for bacterial overgrowth, but this is rarely performed.

Small bowel radiology will usually identify jejunal diverticulum, distal ileal disease, strictures, CD, lymphoma and tumors. CT scanning can also be helpful in lymphoma and looking for carcinoid or other neuroendocrine tumors.

If a pancreatic cause for malabsorption is suspected, investigations are directed to assess the underlying pathology as well as the functional aspect of enzyme deficiency. Pancreatic carcinoma can be difficult to diagnose/differentiate from chronic pancreatitis.

Treatment

Bacterial overgrowth, bile salt malabsorption and carbohydrate intolerance are often treated empirically before embarking on more specific complicated tests. This is in part due to the ease of prescribing treatment and/or high false-positive rates for the tests. Bacterial overgrowth is treated with antibiotics, such as tetracycline, metronidazole, ciprofloxacin and erythromycin. This is given for 2 weeks each, and prolonged cyclical treatment may be necessary. Cholestyramine is used for bile acid malabsorption. The management for carbohydrate intolerance is dietary restriction.

Chronic pancreatitis

The presenting features of chronic pancreatitis consist of abdominal pain, diarrhea due to exocrine deficiency causing malabsorption and, rarely, diabetes mellitus. The pain is typically localized diffusely in the upper abdomen and sometimes radiates to the back. It is usually made worse with eating. The presence of a complication such as an enlarging pseudocyst or ductal obstruction may result in the pain becoming more intense or persistent. The natural history of the pain is variable. Chronic pancreatitis can be painless in 15% of cases and differentiation from pancreatic carcinoma is difficult.

Endocrine insufficiency occurs late, and impaired glucose tolerance and frank diabetes manifests in 30%.

The commonest cause is chronic alcohol abuse (70–80%). Others include gallstones, cystic fibrosis, alpha-1 antitrypsin deficiency and congenital pancreas abnormalities. In a large number, no cause is found.

Plain abdominal X-ray may show ductal calcification in 30% of cases. Abdominal ultrasound may show tumors, cysts and ductal dilatation. The sensitivity and specificity of diagnosis of chronic pancreatitis is 50–70% and 80–90%, respectively. CT is superior to ultrasound for diagnosis (sensitivity 75–90%, specificity > 90%) as well as identifying the complications. ERCP is the most sensitive modality for diagnosis with sensitivity and specificity both in excess of 90%. It can reveal strictures, side-branch dilatation and small calculi. MRCP and endoscopic ultrasound are other imaging techniques being evaluated, and the latter is thought to be comparable to ERCP for diagnosis. Despite all these imaging modalities, the differentiation from pancreatic carcinoma in the absence of vascular invasion is difficult.

Pancreatic exocrine function can be assessed formally but direct and indirect pancreatic function tests are rarely used, as management is rarely altered. Indirect pancreatic function tests are sometimes used to support the radiological findings of probable diagnosis. These include measurement of fecal chymotrypsin or elastase 1, the enzyme actions using the bentiromide (NBT-PABA) test or pancreolauryl test (see *Table 8.3*). The pancreolauryl test may be helpful in distinguishing pancreatic from other causes of steatorrhea. The low sensitivity and specificity, particularly in mild to moderate disease, limit their usefulness in 'screening'.

Management involves adequate analgesia, pancreatic enzyme supplementation and medium-chain triglyceride. If steatorrhea is 'refractory' to optimal enzyme supplementation (> 30 000 units each meal) with acid suppression therapy, patient compliance needs to be assessed. This involves a careful history and consideration of a repeat pancreolauryl test (if abnormal initially). A decrease in fat intake may be necessary. Insulin is usually needed for treatment of diabetes, as oral hypoglycemics are often ineffective. Glycemic control can be difficult and hypoglycemia is common.

Surgery is sometimes used for intractable pain where there is localized chronic pancreatitis or focal lesions. Pseudocysts may require drainage percutaneously or surgically.

Lymphocytic/collagenous colitis

Lymphocytic and collagenous colitis are relatively rare conditions, comprising the microscopic colitides. Despite the similarities in presentation and clinical course, it remains to be established whether the two are separate entities or a variation of the same disease. The diagnosis can be missed unless large bowel biopsies are taken. They usually affect patients over 60 and collagenous colitis is more common in women. Typically, the diarrhea is watery without blood.

Abdominal pain may be present. Routine blood tests are often unremarkable. The colonic mucosa looks normal macroscopically but, histologically, inflammation and lymphocytic/plasma cells' infiltration of the lamina propria is seen. Deposition of a layer of type IV collagen in the subepithelial region of the colonic mucosa is characteristic of collagenous colitis.

Twenty-seven per cent of patients with refractory celiac disease may have microscopic colitis. Five per cent of patients with celiac disease have microscopic colitis. Conversely, 27% of patients with microscopic colitis (lymphocytic > collagenous) have some degree of villous atrophy.

Treatment is empirical with up to 50% response to sulphasalazine. Other 5-ASA agents or steroids can also be used for symptomatic control. Loperamide, antibiotics (e.g. metronidazole, ciprofloxacin) and cholestyramine have all been used with good results. Patients are advised to stop NSAID use.

An approach to a patient with constipation

History

The approach is similar to the patient with chronic diarrhea and many of the generalizations are applicable. For instance, longevity of symptoms is usually associated with a benign cause (*Box 8.3*).

> **Box 8.3 Important factors in history of a patient with constipation**
>
> • Meaning of constipation
> • Duration of symptoms
> • Preceding/precipitating events
> • Associated features
> • Past medical/surgical history
> • Family history
> • Drug history

It is crucial to explore the meaning of constipation. Description of severe straining and difficulty defecating, but normal bowel frequency and stool consistency, is typical of pelvic muscle dysfunction. In the case of constipation, dietary history will be focused on adequacy of fiber and fluid intake. Poor erratic meal intake due to work shifts in certain professions may be relevant. Intermittent constipation alternating with diarrhea or coincidence of symptom onset with stressful life events suggest a functional problem. In the associated features, rectal pain or bleeding suggests a possible cause (e.g. anal fissure) or complication of constipation. Weight loss or anorexia are sinister features that require detailed evaluation. Constipation may present as a feature of another systemic problem such as hypothyroidism.

Past obstetric history of difficult labor/vaginal delivery is particularly relevant for pelvic muscle dysfunction. Look for history of lack of call to stool, call to stool with straining or incomplete evacuation. The relation of symptom to a new drug, such as opioid analgesia, amitriptyline or aluminum-containing antacids, is extremely common. Some patients may admit to a prolonged history of self-medication with stimulant laxatives. A subgroup of patients may have psychosocial problems, including eating disorders or history of sexual abuse.

Table 8.4. Common causes of constipation

Inadequate dietary fiber; dehydration	
Drugs	Opiates; aluminum containing antacids; iron supplements; anticholinergic agents; anti-parkinsonian drugs; tricyclic antidepressants
Functional bowel disorders	
Mechanical problems	
Anorectal disorders	Anal fissure; anal stenosis; hemorrhoids; anterior mucosal prolapse; tumors
Colonic disorders	Strictures from diverticular disease, carcinoma or inflammatory bowel disease
Gynecological	Ovarian and uterine tumors
Endocrine and metabolic	Diabetes mellitus (autonomic neuropathy); hypothyroidism; hypercalcemia, hypokalemia; uremia
Neuromuscular causes	Hirschsprung's disease, autonomic neuropathy, multiple sclerosis, paraplegia; lumbosacral cord/cauda equina trauma or compression; progressive systemic sclerosis
Idiopathic slow transit	

History taking and physical examination should be performed with these disorders in mind (*see Table 8.4*).

Examination

As in assessment for chronic diarrhea, a thorough systematic examination is necessary. This looks for signs of conditions that are associated with constipation, and any sinister features to suggest neoplastic process. Abdominal examination, specifically for any abdominal mass, and a detailed rectal examination for anal tone, masses and fissures are essential.

Investigations and management (*Table 8.5*)

Blood tests will help identify most organic and treatable causes as discussed in the section on investigating diarrhea. Hypercalcemia can cause constipation, and common causes include malignancy and primary hyperparathyroidism.

Table 8.5. Basic investigations for constipation

Blood tests	U&E, thyroid function, glucose, calcium	Exclude diabetes mellitus, hypercalcemia, hypothyroidism
Endoscopy and worrying radiology	Flexible sigmoidoscopy and	If over age 40, with rectal bleeding or other
	barium enema	features, or strong family history of bowel cancer
		Colonoscopy instead if any polyp identified or resources permitting

U&E, urea and electrolytes

Proctoscopy or sigmoidoscopy is indicated particularly in the presence of rectal bleeding. Rectal tumors and the presence of melanosis coli, suggestive of anthraquinone consumption, may be visible. Colonoscopy or flexible sigmoidoscopy with double contrast barium enema should be considered, especially if the patient is over 40 with symptoms of recent onset and colorectal carcinoma is suspected. Surgical referral is needed, particularly for mechanical problems such as repair of rectal/mucosal prolapse. The majority of patients are then treated empirically without further investigations.

Some patients require additional tests for severe symptoms or poor response to dietary and lifestyle changes and/or laxative treatment (*Table 8.6*). Colonic transit studies are useful to document slow transit constipation, and differentiate between diffuse transit problem or segmental/pelvic floor dysfunction. There is, however, a poor correlation between colonic transit time and reported stool frequency, which can be as little as once or twice a fortnight. Idiopathic slow transit causes constipation in young women. Such patients also complain of painful defecation and abdominal discomfort, but are otherwise healthy.

Table 8.6. Specialized investigations for constipation

Radiology	
Colonic transit study	To look for delayed transit, and characterize diffuse or segmental delay/pelvic floor dysfunction Stop any drugs affecting colonic motility
Anorectal manometry	Pelvic muscle dysfunction
Barium defecography	Assessing rectal prolapse, rarely performed
Electromyography	Assessment of incontinence, rarely performed

Transit study involves ingestion of radio-opaque markers while on a high-fiber diet. Plain abdominal X-rays at days 2 and 5 normally show 75–80% excretion by day 5. In idiopathic slow transit, excretion is delayed, and markers may be seen throughout the colon at day 5. In contrast, the markers may move rapidly and then retained in the rectum, indicating megarectum.

Anorectal manometry is indicated to diagnose a neuromuscular cause of constipation, and to confirm pelvic muscle dysfunction before referral for biofeedback therapy. It complements the findings of colonic transit study, especially when surgery is considered. The parameters that can be tested include:

- Anal sphincter function
- Anorectal pressure response to increase in abdominal pressure
- Changes in anal tone during attempted defecation
- Rectal sensation, compliance and motor function
- Recto-anal reflex

Electromyography measures external sphincter and puborectalis muscle activity during attempted defecation. This is useful in assessing pudendal nerve function in patients with fecal incontinence. Barium defecography or defecating proctography assess the mechanics of defecation, including whether the perineum descends, causing a rectal prolapse. This is usually seen after the pudendal nerve is damaged during childbirth.

Idiopathic constipation

Once organic disease has been ruled out and treated appropriately, we are left with a proportion of patients who require management of the symptom itself. Functional bowel disorder/IBS may require psychological assessment and therapy (see Chapter 12). Most patients obtain symptom control or improvement through lifestyle, dietary and pharmacological measures.

Box 8.4	Choice of laxative
Bulk forming	Ispaghula husk (Fybogel®), Celevac®, Normacol®
Osmotic	Magnesium sulfate (Epsom salts), lactulose
Stimulant	Bisacodyl, senna (Senokot®, Manevac®)

Simple general measures such as ensuring an adequate dietary fiber intake and fluid intake should be instituted. Regular exercise and not ignoring a call to stool should also be suggested.

Laxatives can be used, preferably temporarily and at a low dose as needed (*Box 8.4*). A bulk-forming agent such as Fybogel may be effective initially with an increased fluid intake. If this is ineffective, then an osmotic agent such as lactulose should be tried next. Nonfermentable magnesium salts may be preferred if flatulence is a problem. A stimulant laxative such as senna may be helpful, but should be restricted to the short term as there is concern that long-term use may damage the enteric nervous system (cathartic megacolon).

If the constipation appears refractory to treatment, a brief period of inpatient stay for intensive purgative treatment can be arranged. Enemas may be required in constipation causing overflow. The patient with psychiatric symptoms needs referral for psychological evaluation.

Surgery is rarely an option; colonic transit study is essential before considering surgery. Colectomy and ileorectal anastamosis can be used in exceptional cases for idiopathic slow transit.

Pelvic floor dysfunction

Other terminology used for this condition includes dyssynergic or obstructive defecation. The history is characterized by difficulty or inability to expel stools. This is supported by history of difficult labor or perianal trauma during parturition. The investigation of choice is anorectal manometry and/or colonic transit study. It is important to identify these patients, as biofeedback has been shown to be helpful for those with poor coordination between rectum and anus. Visual and verbal feedback techniques are used to achieve anal relaxation, anorectal coordination and sensory conditioning.

Further reading

American Gastroenterological Association medical position statement (1999) Guidelines for the Evaluation and Management of Chronic Diarrhea. *Gastroenterology* **116**: 1461–1463.

American Gastroenterological Association medical position statement (2000) Guidelines on Constipation. *Gastroenterology* **119**: 1761–1778.

Baert, F., Wouters, K., D'Haens, G., *et al.* (1999) Lymphocytic colitis: a distinct clinical entity? A clinicopathological confrontation of lymphocytic and collagenous colitis. *Gut* **45**: 375–381.

Luth, S., Teyssen, S., Forssmann, K., *et al.* (2001) Faecal elastase-1 determination: 'gold' standard of indirect pancreatic function tests? *Scand. J. Gastroenterol.* **36**: 1092–1099.

Plevris, J.N. and Hayes, P.C. (1996–1997) Investigation and management of acute diarrhoea. *Br. J. Hosp. Med.* **56**: 569–573.

Travis, S.P.L., Taylor, R.H. and Misiewicz, J.J. (1998) *Gastroenterology*. Blackwell Scientific, Oxford.

Turnberg, L.A. (1989) *Clinical Gastroenterology*. Blackwell Scientific Publications, Oxford.

Wallace, M.B. and Hawes, R.H. (2001) Endoscopic ultrasound in the evaluation and treatment of chronic pancreatitis. *Pancreas* **23**: 26–35.

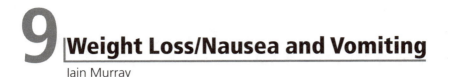

9 Weight Loss/Nausea and Vomiting

Iain Murray

Introduction

Investigation and management of both weight loss and nausea and vomiting can present a great challenge to gastroenterologists. Where they present as one of a number of symptoms, the other symptoms will often help guide investigations. When presenting alone, there are a wide range of conditions that may be responsible, and a comprehensive history and examination are essential. Neither symptom is readily investigated through a diagnostic algorithm, as in other symptom complexes.

Management approach to a patient with weight loss

Initial assessment

Although patients with weight loss as the sole presenting complaint will be referred to a gastroenterologist, not all will have a GI disorder. One-third will have cancer, often of the GI tract, one-quarter will remain unexplained despite extensive investigation and the remainder will have one of a number of chronic diseases, primarily psychiatric or GI (see *Table 9.1*). Of all referrals, one-quarter will die within a year.

As part of the initial assessment, it is important to determine whether the weight loss has been intentional and whether appetite has altered. The amount and duration of the weight loss, together with an idea of whether weight previously had tended to be stable or fluctuate should also be determined. Those with deliberate weight loss often exaggerate the amount lost while those with organic disease will tend to minimize their reported losses. Loss of weight is more likely to be significant when weight has been stable throughout adult life than when it has fluctuated.

Weight loss only occurs when energy expenditure exceeds intake. In most cases, this is a result of anorexia, a loss of the desire to eat (loss of appetite). Increased energy expenditure (due to an increase in physical activity, increase in metabolic activity due to endocrine disorder or malignant cachexia with elevated cytokine expression, including tumor necrosis factor α; TNFα) will result in weight loss unless calorie intake is increased correspondingly. Diarrhea or loss of nutrients in the urine may contribute to this.

Table 9.1. Causes of weight loss

Malignancy	Primarily gastrointestinal: any tumor may present with weight loss

Gastrointestinal disease
  Conditions producing dysphagia
  Early satiety
  Malabsorption
  Fistulae and bypasses, e.g. malignancy,
  Crohn's, celiac disease, esophageal stricture
	
	Nausea/vomiting
	Diarrhea
	Chronic inflammation

Endocrine disorders
  Hyperthyroidism
  Pheochromocytoma
  Hypercalcemia (especially due to malignancy
  but also hyperparathyroidism)
	
	Uncontrolled diabetes mellitus
	Hypoadrenalism (Addison's disease)

Chronic illness	Including HIV, congestive cardiac failure, chronic obstructive pulmonary disease, fever

Psychiatric disorders
  Depression
  Delusion/paranoid disorders
  Bipolar affective disorder – both manic and
  depressive phases
  Neuroleptic withdrawal cachexia – rapid
  tapering or discontinuing chlorpromazine,
  thioridazine, haloperidol
	
	Anorexia nervosa/bulimia
	Munchausen's syndrome

Drug use
  Nicotine
  Opiates
  Fluoxetine and other serotonin re-uptake
  inhibitors
  Levodopa, nonsteroidal anti-inflammatory
  drugs, digoxin, metformin
	
	Amphetamines, cocaine

Investigations

Initial investigations will be determined by history, particularly on changes in appetite. Weight loss with increased appetite occurs only in a few conditions (*Box 9.1*) and therefore a few specific tests should be considered as the first line of investigation (*Box 9.2*).

It is more common to find decreased appetite in association with weight loss, either relating to anorexia or to a fear of provoking discomfort/pain (sitophobia). Drugs that can cause anorexia (see *Table 9.1*) should be stopped where possible. If there are associated symptoms or physical findings, these should guide initial investiga-

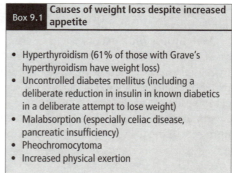

Box 9.1	Causes of weight loss despite increased appetite

- Hyperthyroidism (61% of those with Grave's hyperthyroidism have weight loss)
- Uncontrolled diabetes mellitus (including a deliberate reduction in insulin in known diabetics in a deliberate attempt to lose weight)
- Malabsorption (especially celiac disease, pancreatic insufficiency)
- Pheochromocytoma
- Increased physical exertion

tions. Otherwise, minimum screening tests are listed in *Box 9.3*.

Although 42% of the patients with Grave's hyperthyroidism have increased appetite, more have weight loss with normal or decreased appetite ('apathetic' hyperthyroidism), especially the elderly.

Box 9.2	Investigations for weight loss with normal or increased appetite

- Thyroid function tests
- Random blood glucose
- IgA endomysial antibody titers and total IgA
- 24-h urinary vanillylmondelic acid (VMA) (following appropriate dietary exclusions)
- Indirect tests of exocrine pancreatic function, e.g. pancreolauryl test, NBT-PABA test, fecal-elastase-1 or fecal chymotrypsin

Weight loss with hyperthyroidism can be substantial, averaging 16% in one series. If hypoadrenalism is considered, a short Synacthen test should be performed. HIV testing must not be performed without adequate counseling and consent from the patient. This should be documented in their case notes.

Box 9.3	Investigations for weight loss with decreased appetite

- Urea and electrolytes
- Liver function tests
- Serum calcium
- Glucose
- Thyroid function tests
- Full blood count
- IgA endomysial antibodies and total IgA level
- Inflammatory markers (CRP, ESR)
- Chest X-ray

Despite intensive investigation, a diagnosis is not found in up to a quarter of those presenting with weight loss alone. A dietetic assessment of calorie intake can be helpful, especially when corroborated by family or friends. Generally, it is obvious when a psychiatric disorder underlies the weight loss, but sensitive probing may reveal depression, anorexia nervosa or very rarely Munchausen's syndrome.

Management

The optimum management of weight loss is identification and treatment of the underlying condition. Profound weight loss can be seen even in benign conditions and may be associated with vitamin and mineral deficiencies. Early dietetic assessment and support is vital, with the aims of not only preventing further weight loss but also recovering lost calories. Vitamin and mineral deficiencies should be sought and replacement therapy given when necessary. Deficiencies of folate, B_{12}, iron and magnesium can lead to mouth ulceration and altered taste, which can exacerbate the reduced calorie intake.

Management approach to a patient with nausea and vomiting

Defining the problem

Like weight loss, nausea and vomiting can have many causes, not all GI in origin. The need for investigation and likelihood of major pathology is based on careful assessment of symptoms and associated features together with clinical examination.

Nausea is defined as the unpleasant sensation of the imminent need to vomit, vomiting being the forceful expulsion of gastric contents associated with the contraction of respiratory and abdominal muscles. Its physiological function is to rid the body of potentially harmful toxins. Retching is the spasmodic contraction of respiratory muscles, with abdominal muscle contraction against a closed glottis so that there is no expulsion of gastric contents. Regurgitation involves bringing food back into the mouth without the forceful abdominal and respiratory muscle contraction, which may occur voluntarily during the act of eating or shortly afterwards as in rumination. Chronic nausea and vomiting is defined arbitrarily as lasting more than 1 month. Acute nausea and vomiting is most commonly due to infection, both viral and bacterial gastroenteritis, hepatitis, meningitis, pancreatitis, cholecystitis and otitis media, motion sickness or drugs. The cause is usually obvious, the course self-limiting by definition and hence unlikely to result in referral to a GI outpatient department. It will not be considered further here.

Management of nausea and vomiting requires recognition of the consequences of vomiting, determination of the underlying causes and control of the symptoms where necessary.

Recognition of consequences

Frequent and prolonged episodes of vomiting can result in fluid and electrolyte disturbance, particularly hypokalemic metabolic alkalosis, sometimes with vitamin and trace element deficiencies. Clinical evidence of hypovolemia (tachycardia, postural drop in blood pressure and increase in pulse rate) merits urgent admission for intravenous fluid replacement. U&Es, including serum bicarbonate, should be checked in all patients with vomiting, and vitamin and mineral levels in those with a protracted course.

Clinical assessment

There are many causes of nausea and vomiting (see *Box 9.4*) making evaluation of the patient presenting with these symptoms seemingly impossible. However, a careful and complete history and examination will often help to elicit the likely cause and therefore the most appropriate investigations.

Differentiation of vomiting from regurgitation and rumination is essential. Regurgitation is passive without the violent abdominal and respiratory muscle contractions seen with vomiting. It generally begins during or within minutes of eating, is not preceded by nausea or retching and the regurgitated food does not taste bitter or acid.

The duration, frequency and severity of vomiting should be determined. Chronic nausea and vomiting (> 1 month duration) is further explored here. Vomiting in the morning is characteristic of pregnancy, raised intracranial pressure, alcohol excess and uremia. That due to raised intracranial pressure is classically 'projectile'.

Box 9.4	Causes of nausea and vomiting

Acute (defined as lasting < 4 weeks)	*Chronic*
Gastroenteritis – viral, bacterial, parasitic	Pyloric stenosis – benign or malignant
Exogenous toxins	Gastroesophageal reflux
Endocrine	Gastroparesis
Pregnancy	Viral
Uremia	Diabetic
Diabetic ketoacidosis	Paraneoplastic
Hyperparathyroidism	Idiopathic
Hypoparathyroidism	Intestinal obstruction
Thyrotoxicosis	Eosinophilic gastroenteritis
Addison's disease	Chronic intestinal pseudo-obstruction
Labyrinthitis	Cyclic vomiting syndrome
Raised intracranial pressure	Rumination syndrome
Postoperative vomiting	Bulimia
Postchemotherapy	Functional/psychogenic vomiting
Drugs including opiate analgesia, digoxin, L-dopa,	Starvation
bromocriptine, nicotine, non-steroidal anti-inflammatory	Any of causes listed under 'acute', especially
drugs, sulfasalazine, oral hypoglycemic agents and	endocrine causes, neurogenic, drugs
many others	
Jamaican vomiting sickness (unripe akee fruit)	

If there is esophageal pathology, such as a stricture, diverticulum or achalasia, vomiting occurs soon after eating and the foodstuff is recognizable. Regurgitation rather than vomiting may be seen. Vomiting due to gastric outlet obstruction or gastroparesis typically occurs an hour or more after eating. The food is partly digested. Small bowel obstruction results in bilious or feculent vomitus.

Coexistent symptoms will also aid in the diagnosis. Abdominal pain particularly preceding vomiting is usually due to organic GI pathology, including intestinal obstruction.

Weight loss can be due to malignancy or benign gastric outlet obstruction. Important details in the history are fever (gastroenteritis, viral gastroparesis), diarrhea (gastroenteritis), whether others have been affected (gastroenteritis) and whether there is vertigo (labyrinthitis, cerebral pathology). A neurological history should be elicited, especially headache, vertigo and any focal neurological deficit.

Gastroparesis can cause early satiety, postprandial fullness, bloating and pain, especially in females. Early satiety can also be a symptom of gastric malignancy.

Physical examination should concentrate on excluding hypovolemia, and looking for abdominal masses, herniae, jaundice or lymphadenopathy. Abdominal distention, visible peristalsis and succussion splash suggest obstruction, especially with increased bowel sounds. Signs of Addison's disease and thyrotoxicosis should be sought and a full neurological examination performed. Hands must be examined for signs of scleroderma or peripheral neuropathy and the dorsum for calluses (seen in bulimia). Dental enamel is lost in bulimia and occasionally in severe GERD.

Investigations

Basic investigations include full blood count, U&Es, inflammatory markers, thyroid-stimulating hormone and a pregnancy test in menstruating women. Drug levels in patients taking digoxin, theophylline or salicylates should be determined. Addison's disease should be excluded where there is any clinical suspicion (including hyponatremia and postural hypotension).

Further investigations are dependent upon initial assessment. In some patients without 'sinister' features, a therapeutic trial of antiemetics may be indicated. A cost-benefit analysis of this approach has not been performed. Where GI pathology is suspected, an upper GI endoscopy is preferable to a barium meal. It is more sensitive for the detection of minor mucosal abnormalities, permits biopsies for histological confirmation of tumor, allows gastric biopsies to exclude the rare condition of eosinophilic gastroenteritis (peripheral eosinophilia in two-thirds, history of atopy in half) and involves no radiation exposure. However, it is more expensive than barium meal studies, and has the risks of complications associated with the procedure (hemorrhage, perforation) and with sedation where used.

Where intestinal obstruction is suspected, a plain abdominal X-ray can be helpful. Small bowel enema is more sensitive than small bowel follow-through study for the detection of small tumors, although it requires the placement of a nasoduodenal or oroduodenal tube into the small bowel. A CT scan of the abdomen after oral and intravenous contrast may be more sensitive still, and detects pathology of the pancreas, hepatobiliary system, urogenital tracts and retroperitoneum.

The role of studies of gastric motor function is unclear. They can be useful to confirm a clinical suspicion of gastroparesis, but often do not result in changes in therapy. The most common of these tests is the radionuclide gastric-emptying study, most sensitive using solid-phase meals. The radiation exposure is twice that from a plain abdominal X-ray. Delayed emptying is typically seen in gastroparesis, but this neither proves that this is the cause of symptoms nor determines the underlying cause of the gastroparesis.

Electrogastrography and antroduodenal manometry are offered in some tertiary centers. Electrogastrography uses similar monitoring electrodes to those for electrocardiography to record gastric resting motor activity and the response to food. Gastric brady- and tachycardia can be seen in gastroparesis, nausea from pregnancy and motion sickness, and no increase in motor activity is typically seen in gastroparesis. Antroduodenal manometry records directly through intraluminal pressure transducers and again can measure motor activity in fasting and postprandial states. Antral hypomotility is frequently seen in unexplained nausea and vomiting. Unfortunately, its finding rarely results in changes in therapy. Occasionally changes of chronic intestinal pseudo-obstruction or even mechanical obstruction may be seen with antroduodenal manometry when not previously suspected. It may be useful when other tests have been negative, to completely exclude gastroparesis or GI obstruction.

Intracranial imaging is best performed by MRI rather than CT because of superior images of the posterior fossa. It is very rare to find intracranial space occupying lesions in adults, causing nausea and vomiting in the absence of a history of headache and with a normal neurological examination.

Psychological evaluation can be helpful to exclude depression, anxiety, hysteria and hypochondriasis once organic pathology has been excluded.

Management

The first step in management should be fluid and electrolyte replacement using normal saline with potassium supplements where required.

Frequent small meals with reduction in fat content, and avoidance of indigestible foodstuffs and carbonated drinks, can sometimes help in gastroparesis. Gastric pacing has been used where this and pharmacological measures have failed. Where drugs may be the underlying cause of nausea and vomiting, these should be discontinued. Drugs usually cause symptoms soon after their commencement rather than when they have been used for some time.

Drugs used to control nausea and vomiting are either antiemetics, which are centrally acting or prokinetics (see *Table 9.2*). It is often easier to control and prevent vomiting than nausea.

Behavioral therapy can benefit those with regurgitation and rumination.

Table 9.2. Pharmacological agents used in the management of nausea and vomiting

Class of drug	Examples	Indications	Common side-effects
Antiemetics			
Antihistamines (H1)	Meclozine (PO), dramamine (PO), cyclizine (PO, im, iv), cinnarizine (PO), promethazine (PO)	Motion sickness, vertigo, migraine	Drowsiness, dry mouth, blurred vision
Phenothiazines	Prochlorperazine (PO, im, pr), chlorpromazine (PO, im, pr), perphenazine (PO), trifluoperazine (PO)	Severe nausea and vomiting (all), vertigo, labyrinthitis (prochlorperazine only)	Extrapyramidal side-effects, especially dystonic reactions, drowsiness, blood dyscrasias (trifluoperazine)
Serotonin (5-HT) antagonists	Ondansetron (PO, iv, im, pr), granisetron (PO, iv), tropisetron (PO, iv, im)	Cytotoxic chemotherapy, radiotherapy, post-operative	Constipation, headache, rash, elevated liver enzymes, hypersensitivity
Substituted benzamides	Domperidone (PO, pr), metoclopramide (PO, im, iv)	Nausea/vomiting including drug-induced, post-operative, chemotherapy	Hyperprolactinemia, extrapyramidal effects (metoclopramide)
Cannabinoids	Nabilone (PO)	Cytotoxic chemotherapy	Drowsiness, vertigo, euphoria, dry mouth, ataxia, visual disturbance, sleep disturbance, concentration difficulties
Prokinetics			
Substituted benzamides	As above		
Macrolide	Erythromycin (iv)	Although has prokinetic effects, not licensed in UK for this indication	Nausea, vomiting, diarrhea, abdominal discomfort, allergic reactions

im, intramuscular; iv, intravenous; PO, orally; pr, per rectum

Nausea and vomiting – difficult problems

Gastroparesis (including that in diabetes mellitus)

Management of gastroparesis should deal with maintaining adequate nutrition and hydration, ensuring optimum diabetic control, medical therapy and occasionally surgery, including gastric electrical stimulation.

As well as fluid losses, hypokalemia, metabolic acidosis and iron and B_{12} deficiencies need to be replenished. If oral diet is possible, this should be liquidized or homogenized and should avoid high fat and fiber content. If oral replacement is not possible, then jejunal feeding should be attempted. A trial of nasojejunal feeding is appropriate before proceeding to jejunostomy via laparotomy or through a percutaneous gastrostomy. The patient should be able to tolerate a feed rate of 80 ml h^{-1} if they are to be adequately hydrated and nourished by this means. Occasionally parenteral feeding is required.

Better glycemic control may improve gastric emptying, although this has not been conclusively proven. Certainly gastric stasis can affect glycemic control. Dietary modifications, including small meals frequently, low fiber and fat and homogenized or liquid meals, may increase gastric emptying.

Intravenous erythromycin (3 mg kg^{-1} tds) can be helpful during acute episodes of gastric stasis, but oral administration is less effective and there is the risk of GI toxicity, ototoxicity and pseudomembranous colitis with long-term use. Cisapride 10–20 mg four times daily stimulates antral and duodenal motility but can produce diarrhea. However, it has been withdrawn from use in the UK, the USA and much of Europe because of cardiac arrhythmias, especially torsade de pointes, especially when administered to those with prolonged QT interval on electrocardiogram (ECG), with macrolide antibiotics, antifungals and phenothiazines, and at doses greater than 1 mg kg^{-1} day^{-1}. It may be obtainable on compassionate grounds and on a named patient basis from the manufacturers. Metoclopramide both orally and intravenously and oral domperidone can be used. Metoclopramide has the rare side-effect of tardive dyskinesia and anxiety, restlessness and depression.

Percutaneous or laparoscopically placed gastrostomy or jejunostomy tubes can be used to decompress the upper gut. Surgery is rarely necessary otherwise, although patients with gastroparesis following partial gastrectomy may be offered subtotal or total gastrectomy and gastrojejunostomy. A significant improvement in symptoms following surgery is seen in two-thirds.

Experimentally, gastric electric stimulation at 12 counts per minute (four times greater than the intrinsic slow wave activity) has been shown to be of some benefit. At present, the use of these devices has been approved in the USA in approved centers in chronically ill patients with refractory idiopathic and diabetic gastroparesis.

Chronic intestinal pseudo-obstruction

Again, nutritional support and prokinetics including metoclopramide, erythromycin and cisapride (with the above proviso) are the mainstays of therapy. Antibiotics (rotating courses of ciprofloxacin, doxycycline and metronidazole for example) can be used if there is documented small bowel bacterial overgrowth. Subcutaneous octreotide improves intestinal pseudo-obstruction both idiopathic and that due to scleroderma. Neostigmine has been used in acute but not chronic intestinal pseudo-obstruction. Surgical resection of localized disease in the small intestine, or of the colon when chronic constipation results in chronic pseudo-obstruction, may be necessary.

Bulimia nervosa

A multidisciplinary team approach should be adopted, with a minimum of medical, nutritional and mental health carers. The role of the medical carer is to manage physical problems, including fluid and electrolyte disturbance, and to act as coordinator of care. A dietician will work with the patient to provide nutritional education and define appropriate goals, and the mental health provider will provide the psychological treatment, usually cognitive behavioral therapy.

Reasonable goals for weight gain in outpatients with eating disorders are 0.25–0.5 kg per week, whereas inpatients should be able to achieve gains of 1–1.5 kg per week, commencing initially with a calorie intake of 1000–1600 kcal day^{-1} and increasing. Cognitive behavioral therapy is the most effective psychotherapy for bulimia, helping patients to recognize the disordered thought processes that result in their eating disorder and allowing them to develop coping strategies. Fluoxetine, desipramine, imipramine, amitriptyline, monoamine oxidase inhibitors and buspirone have all been shown to reduce binge eating and vomiting in bulimia.

The decision to hospitalize patients with eating disorders should be based on medical, psychiatric and behavioral criteria. Weight less than 75% of ideal body weight should prompt admission with discharge delayed until body weight is 90–92% ideal. Early discharge results in poorer long-term outcome. Admission may be to medical or psychiatric wards according to patient condition and local resources.

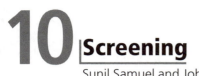

10 | Screening

Sunil Samuel and John Wong

Introduction

Screening is becoming an important part of the work of a gastroenterologist. This trend is likely to continue over the next 10–15 years as the evidence, particularly with respect to colorectal cancer, emerges.

Criteria for screening are:

- The condition should be common
- The condition should be an important problem in the community
- There should be an effective treatment for the condition
- The cost of the screening procedure must be cost effective
- The screening test should be accurate and acceptable to the patients

Colorectal cancer screening

Colorectal cancer is the second commonest cause of cancer related death in the developed world with an average 5-year survival of 40%. In the UK approximately 20 000 deaths are due to colorectal cancer. It is typically asymptomatic in the early stages and hence the majority of cases are detected at a relatively advanced stage (Dukes B–D), which adversely affects survival. Patients with early colon cancer (Dukes A) have a 5-year survival of 90% compared to 64%, 38%, and 3% for Dukes B, C and D, respectively.

Several studies have now confirmed that adequate screening programs improve survival in patients with colorectal cancer by detecting cancers at an early stage. However, although all the major studies have shown improved survival, the optimal screening methods remain a matter of debate.

The biology of colorectal cancer lends itself to early detection by screening. The majority of colorectal cancers arise in adenomatous polyps, and removal of these polyps reduces the subsequent incidence of cancer. However, polyps are no more common in patients with hereditary nonpolyposis colon cancer (HNPCC) than in the general population. The method and timing of screening vary, depending on the individual patient's risk of developing colorectal cancer. It is therefore vital for clinicians to decide whether the individual is at high, medium or low risk (see *Box 10.1*). A few simple questions would help to stratify an individual's risk of colorectal cancer:

- Is there a family history of colorectal cancer? If so, whether in first-degree relatives, their age of onset and how many
- Past history of colorectal cancer or adenomatous polyps

Low-risk group

One first-degree relative with colorectal cancer > 55 years

No family history of colorectal cancer (general population)

Medium-risk group

People with large (> 1 cm) or multiple adenomatous polyps of any size

Personal history of curative-intent resection of colorectal cancer

One first-degree relative with colorectal cancer < 55 years

Two or more first-degree relatives of any age with colorectal cancer

High-risk group

Familial adenomatous polyposis

Hereditary nonpolyposis colon cancer

Chronic inflammatory bowel disease (≥ 8 years duration, extensive)

- Chronic inflammatory bowel conditions like ulcerative colitis or Crohn's disease

Familial syndromes like HNPCC (*Box 10.2*) and familial adenomatous polyposis (FAP) are associated with an approximately 70% and nearly 100%, respectively, lifetime risk of developing colorectal cancer.

Patients with HNPCC account for 2–5% of all colon cancers. The cancer tends to occur relatively early in life (early 40s). The cancers are more likely to be in the proximal rather than the distal colon. These may be associated with other cancers including cancer of the endometrium, small bowel, ureter or renal pelvis. Polyps are no more common in these patients than the general population.

FAP is characterized by hundreds to thousands of polyps occurring throughout the colon, beginning in adolescence. It is an autosomal dominant disease caused by mutations in the adenomatous polyposis coli (APC) gene, which is located on chromosome 5q21–q22. This accounts for 1% of all colon cancers with tumors developing in the 20s.

IBD affecting the large bowel is associated with increased risk of colorectal cancer, particularly when the disease is long standing (≥ 8 years) and extensive (pancolitis).

Population screening

In a population-screening program, uptake of the offer of the screening test is very important. A survey in the early 1990s showed that the awareness of bowel cancer in the British population was only 30%. This makes the early detection of colorectal cancer more difficult.

The screening tests currently available to detect colorectal cancer are:

- Fecal occult blood test
- Flexible sigmoidoscopy
- Double contrast barium enema
- Colonoscopy
- CT colography (virtual colonoscopy)

Digital rectal examination and rigid sigmoidoscopy are no

Box 10.2	Amsterdam Criteria I for the diagnosis of hereditary nonpolyposis colon cancer

- Three or more relatives with histologically verified colorectal cancer; one of whom is a first-degree relative of the other two; familial adenomatous polyposis excluded
- Colorectal cancer involving at least two generations
- One or more colorectal cases diagnosed before the age of 50

longer considered effective screening methods, as they only detect less than 10% of colorectal cancers.

In spite of the numerous available modalities for population screening, the optimal method and timing are still debated. One of the greatest concerns is the potential damage done to asymptomatic individuals undergoing invasive screening tests. Annual fecal occult blood is probably the most cost effective.

Annual fecal occult blood testing

Several large randomized controlled studies (Nottingham and Minnesota) have now confirmed the effectiveness of annual fecal occult blood testing and mortality reduction of up to 33% has been quoted. A positive test should be followed up by examination of the entire colon with a double contrast barium enema or colonoscopy. The main criticisms were patient compliance and that only 2% of the positive tests had colorectal cancer. Therefore, for every patient with cancer, 50 patients were subjected to unnecessary procedures and anxiety.

Flexible sigmoidoscopy

A large multi-center trial for population screening using once only flexible sigmoidoscopy is underway and results of this should be available in 2003. There is evidence from well-designed, case-controlled studies that flexible sigmoidoscopy reduces mortality by 50–60%. Although flexible sigmoidoscopy is more expensive compared to rigid sigmoidoscopy, it has a much higher yield and is generally more acceptable to the patients. It can easily be performed without sedation and carries much less risk than colonoscopy. More importantly, nurse endoscopists are increasingly performing this procedure, which can make this technique more cost effective.

Screening for medium-risk groups

Patients with large (> 1 cm) or multiple adenomatous polyps

Adenomatous polyps found at flexible sigmoidoscopy should be followed up by colonoscopy to assess the proximal colon. Further polyps, if detected, should be removed. These people should be offered a repeat colonoscopy in 3 years' time and then 5-yearly thereafter.

Patients with a personal history of colorectal cancer

These people, if possible, should have full visualization of the colon at the time of diagnosis to exclude synchronous cancers and polyps, and a subsequent colonoscopy within 1 year of resection and thereafter 3–5-yearly. There is no clear evidence that this affects outcome.

People with family history of colorectal cancer

The inherited risk of colorectal cancer in people with first-degree relatives suffering from colorectal cancer is shown in *Table 10.1*. Total colonic examination, either by colonoscopy or double contrast barium enema, should be offered to all persons with a family history of colorectal cancer in a first-degree relative aged less than 45 or in more than one first-degree relative of any age. The screening should begin at age 40 or 10 years prior to the index case, whichever is early.

Table 10.1. Lifetime risks for colorectal cancer

Family history	Lifetime risk
No family history	1:50
One 1st-degree relative > 45 years	1:18
One 1st-degree relative < 45 years	1:10
Two 1st-degree relatives	1:6

Screening for high-risk groups

Persons with a family history of hereditary nonpolyposis colon cancer

These individuals should be considered for 1–3-yearly colonoscopies, starting between 20 and 25 years of age. Also important is genetic counseling and genetic testing for microsatellite instability (MSI) and germline mutations of the DNA mismatch repair genes. Screening for other associated malignancies is controversial.

Persons with a family history of familial adenomatous polyposis

These people should be offered genetic testing after counseling to identify gene carriers. All carriers of the gene mutation and indeterminate cases should be offered yearly flexible sigmoidoscopy, beginning at puberty, to assess if they are expressing the gene. Sigmoidoscopic examination usually suffices, as the polyps invariably involve the entire colon. Once polyps are detected, the patient should be considered for proctocolectomy, which is the only feasible way to prevent cancer. The American Society for Gastrointestinal Endoscopy also recommends screening and surveillance of the upper GI tract, because of the high risk of cancers of the proximal small bowel.

Patients with chronic inflammatory bowel disease

Patients with pancolitis, due either to ulcerative colitis or CD, are often offered 1–2-yearly surveillance colonoscopies to detect dysplasia. This usually starts at 10 years after diagnosis. There is little objective evidence that this improves prognosis, but it is widely practiced.

Surveillance for dysplasia in Barrett's esophagus

Barrett's esophagus is the replacement of the normal squamous lining of the distal esophageal mucosa with circumferential columnar mucosa containing specialized intestinal epithelium. It is probably the end-result of long-standing reflux disease.

It is well known that Barrett's esophagus is premalignant with the risk of esophageal cancer being 30–120 times higher than the general population. It is presumed that esophageal adenocarcinoma evolves through a multistep process starting from metaplasia through low- and high-grade dysplasia to intramucosal and invasive carcinoma. Several case-controlled studies have shown improved 5-year survival in surveyed patients.

In spite of this understanding, the surveillance endoscopies for patients with Barrett's esophagus remain controversial. The prime reasons for this are:

- The natural history of the disease is unclear
- The true incidence of Barrett's esophagus in the population is likely to be very small
- A survival benefit has not been demonstrated in several randomized, controlled trials
- Endoscopic surveillance is costly

The incidence of adenocarcinoma of the esophagus has risen very rapidly over the last 10–15 years. It is probable that this is because of the increased incidence of Barrett's esophagus. Although there is no strong evidence that screening patients is either cost effective or improves survival, it is difficult to deny screening to patients who are young and have a long segment of affected esophagus. In the UK, there are some well-established screening programs for Barrett's surveillance but many gastroenterology units have had difficulty obtaining the funding for such programs from their local health authorities.

The following recommendations are made by the American College of Gastroenterology:

- Patients not fit for esophagectomy should be excluded from surveillance
- Multiple four-quadrant biopsies should be taken every 2 cm of the Barrett's mucosa
- No dysplasia detected – surveillance endoscopies repeated every 2–3 years
- Low grade dysplasia present – two 6-monthly and then yearly endoscopies
- High grade dysplasia present – esophageal resection should be considered

The place of chromoendoscopy, magnification endoscopy, endoscopic ultra-sound and fluorescence endoscopy in screening patients with Barrett's esophagus remains to be determined.

Screening for hepatocellular carcinoma

The surveillance of patients at risk of hepatocellular carcinoma remains a contentious issue from the viewpoint of cost effectiveness, since an improvement in survival has not been consistently demonstrated.

The patients at risk of hepatocellular cancer are all cirrhotics and chronic carriers of the hepatitis B surface antigen.

Our current practice is to offer all these individuals screening for hepatocellular cancer by 6-monthly AFP and ultrasound of the abdomen. AFP alone is less effective than ultrasound in screening cirrhotics. A study from Hong Kong has shown that patients who underwent screening had smaller cancers and were more amenable to resection.

Screening for hemochromatosis

Family screening

It is generally accepted that first-degree relatives of patients with genetic hemochromatosis should be screened for the disease. Various screening strategies have been used but the most cost-effective method is not clear.

Our current practice is to offer screening for first-degree family members of the proband by fasting transferrin saturation and ferritin estimations with confirmation by genetic testing for HFE gene mutations (C282Y and H63D). The optimal time to initiate screening for family members would be between 18 and 30 years, when hemochromatosis will usually be evident on iron studies but the iron load is not big enough to have caused organ damage. Relatives negative for HFE gene mutations should have follow-up iron studies, as approximately 5% of cases will have the negative gene.

Population screening

Population screening for hemochromatosis is not well established. It may be worthwhile, as the approximate prevalence of hemochromatosis in the general population is 1–4% and the fact that early detection and treatment improves survival. However, the appropriate method and timing of tests is not known.

Genetic testing is not considered cost effective for this type of screening. Routine testing of fasting serum transferrin saturation can be considered but further studies are needed to demonstrate objective evidence.

Further reading

Bacon, B.R. (2001) Haemochromatosis: diagnosis and management. *Gastroenterology* **120**: 718–725.

Bond, J.H. (2000) Polyp guideline: diagnosis, treatment and surveillance for patients with colorectal polyps. *Am. J. Gastroenterol.* **95**: 3053–3063.

Colorectal cancer screening in the UK: Joint Position Statement by the BSG, the Royal Colleges of Physicians & the Association of Coloproctology of Great Britain and Ireland (2001) *Gut* **46**: 746–748.

Pech, O., Gossner, L., May, A. and Ell, C. (2001) Management of Barrett's oesophagus, dysplasia, and early adenocarcinoma. *Best Pract. Res. Clin. Gastroenterol.* **15**: 267–284.

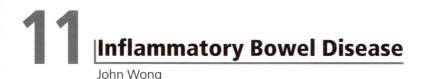

11 Inflammatory Bowel Disease

John Wong

Epidemiology

IBDs consisting of Crohn's disease (CD) and ulcerative colitis (UC) affect up to 0.3% of the UK population. The incidence is estimated to be seven new cases per 100 000 per year for CD, and 11 per 100 000 per year for UC. Both CD and UC have a bimodal age distribution for the onset of disease. Peak incidence for age of onset is 20–30 years for both CD and UC, with a smaller secondary peak at 60–80 years of age.

Pathophysiology

The etiology of IBD remains uncertain. They are thought to be multifactorial diseases caused by interplay of patient factors, such as genetic predisposition and environmental factors. CD and UC are probably related heterogenous polygenic disorders. The mechanisms of inflammation in the gut mucosa are emerging but the cause(s) remains elusive.

Familial prevalence studies and twin concordance data support the evidence for genetic susceptibility to IBD, particularly in CD. A study of IBD from Denmark showed first-degree relatives had a 10-fold increase in the risk of having the same disease as the patient (Orholm *et al.*, 1991). A study from Oxford showed about 13% of patients with CD had an affected relative, most commonly the siblings (Satsangi *et al.*, 1994).

CD can affect the GI tract anywhere from mouth to anus. The most common sites of involvement for CD are terminal ileum and/or cecum (45%), ileocolonic (13%) or colorectal only in about 30%. Rectal involvement is noted at endoscopy in about a third of patients, and this is more prevalent for those with isolated colonic disease. The pattern of presentation for CD can be subclassified into inflammatory, fibrostenotic (stricturing) or fistulating types, which influence the presenting symptoms and clinical outcomes.

UC can similarly be subdivided according to site of involvement into pancolitis, distal colitis or ulcerative proctitis. The disease may progress with time in those patients who are initially diagnosed with distal colitis.

Major extraintestinal manifestations for IBD including sacroiliitis, ankylosing spondylitis and sclerosing cholangitis do not relate to activity of intestinal inflammation. Pyoderma gangrenosum and iritis/uveitis in IBD display some correlation to disease activity. Peripheral large joint arthropathy, stomatitis, and erythema nodosum strongly correspond with activity of intestinal inflammation.

Other complications of IBD include oxalate kidney stones and gallstones (more common in CD), thromboembolism, osteoporosis and amyloidosis. PSC should be suspected in patients who develop abnormal liver biochemical tests.

Diagnosis

Diarrhea and pain are the two most common presenting symptoms for CD. Systemic symptoms such as lethargy, anorexia, weight loss and fever may be present in some patients. The diagnosis may be delayed due to variable symptoms and the often insidious onset of the disease. Abdominal pain symptoms are common in the presence of ileocolonic disease. This may be secondary to underlying inflammatory or fibrostenotic process or adhesions. Right iliac fossa pain, which occurs within 30 min of meals and recurs 3–4 h later, suggests terminal ileal disease. Fistulating disease, including enterocutaneous, internal and perianal fistula, is associated with symptoms such as pneumaturia and abscess-related complications.

Typical presenting symptoms for UC include bloody diarrhea with mucus. Lower abdominal pain, urgency and tenesmus are also common symptoms. At presentation, the majority of patients have mild to moderate disease.

There is a positive association between smoking and CD. One case-control study showed a relative risk of 4.0 in smokers compared to nonsmokers, and suggested a dose-dependent effect (Franceschi *et al.*, 1987). In contrast, studies on smoking habits showed negative association between smoking and UC. There is increased risk of UC among lifelong nonsmokers and exsmokers compared with current smokers. A meta-analysis showed an odds ratio of 0.41 for current smokers compared with lifelong nonsmokers (Calkins, 1989). Appendicectomy has been shown to be another confounding factor that reduces the lifetime risk of UC.

Differential diagnoses and investigations

The main differential diagnoses for the peak of age incidence in the younger age group include infective diarrhea or IBS. For the minor peak of age incidence in the older patients, one needs to consider diverticular disease, ischemic colitis or colon cancer. The sequence of diagnostic investigations may be variable, as determined by presenting symptoms, physical findings and basic laboratory abnormalities (see *Table 11.1*).

Differentiating between Crohn's disease and ulcerative colitis

There are some factors that help to differentiate IBDs. Differentiation can be difficult when CD is limited to the colon, especially in the setting of acute presentation with severe fulminant colitis (see *Table 11.2*).

Table 11.1. Investigations for inflammatory bowel disease (IBD)

	Tests	Rationale
Blood tests	CRP, ESR, thyroid function, endomysial antibody	Exclude hyperthyroidism, celiac disease; raised inflammatory markers support diagnosis of IBD and differentiate from functional bowel conditions
Stool	Microscopy and culture	Rule out infectious diarrhea
Endoscopy	Rigid or flexible sigmoidoscopy or colonoscopy	(1) Terminal ileoscopy, macroscopic appearance and distribution of ulcer lesions, and random colonic biopsies to confirm diagnosis and differentiate between CD or UC (2) Assessment of colitis activity (3) Biopsies from abnormal looking areas or strictures to identify dysplasia or cancer
Radiology	Small bowel barium studies	(1) Look for small bowel/terminal ileum involvement in CD (2) Assessment for post-op recurrent CD, especially if suggestive story of subacute obstruction
Radiology	Ultrasound and CT scan	Delineate and discriminate intra-abdominal masses/abscesses, defining the anatomy and extent of fistula tracks
	MR scan	Direct multiplanar imaging particularly useful in perianal complications

CRP, C-reactive protein; ESR, erythrocyte sedimentation rate; CD, Crohn's disease; UC, ulcerative colitis; CT, computed tomography; MR, magnetic resonance.

Table 11.2. Factors helpful in differentiating between CD and UC

	Tests	Details
Blood tests	p-ANCA and ASCA	p-ANCA is present in about 70% of UC and 15% of CD. ASCA has 67% sensitivity and 92% specificity for CD. These tests are of limited use in everyday practice
Radiology	Small bowel barium studies	Terminal ileum or small bowel involvement is consistent with diagnosis of CD
Endoscopy	Colonoscopy	In UC, diffuse erythema, friability and granularity of mucosa, without skip areas, and rectum always involved
		In CD, rectum is often spared. Aphthous or deeper serpiginous ulcers are seen and typically, skip areas of normal mucosa are seen
Colonic biopsies	Histology	An acute inflammatory reaction with neutrophil infiltrate, crypt abscesses and goblets cells depleted of mucus is supportive of diagnosis of UC. The histology changes are confined to mucosa and submucosa.
		A predominantly lymphocytic infiltrate with transmural involvement is more typical of CD. Submucosal noncaseating granulomata, when present, is a more specific feature.

p-ANCA, perinuclear antineutrophil cytoplasmic antibodies; ASCA, anti-*Saccharomyces cerevisiae* antibody; UC, ulcerative colitis; CD, Crohn's disease.

General management approach for inflammatory bowel diseases

Education

CD and UC are chronic lifelong conditions. Newly diagnosed patients should be offered the opportunity to find out as much as they wish about their condition. It is helpful for the patients to understand the spectrum of disease manifestation and the rationale for long-term use of maintenance therapy. The National Association for Colitis and Crohn's Disease (NACC) is a national organization in the UK that provides good authoritative impartial information. For an annual subscription fee, members receive a pack of information booklets and a quarterly newsletter, plus confidential one-to-one telephone support provided by trained NACC-in-contact volunteers is available. Other information sources include the IBD Club and the Digestive Disorders Foundation (DDF) and no membership fee is required (*Box 11.1*). The meetings of local patient groups not only serve to educate but also to support the psychosocial well-being of patients. A better knowledge of the disease allows the patient to become actively involved in the management decision process together with healthcare professionals.

Box 11.1	Helpful contacts for information on IBD
NACC	The National Association for Colitis and Crohn's Disease (NACC), 4 Beaumont House, Sutton Road, St Albans, Hertfordshire, AL1 5HH; www.nacc.org.uk
DDF	Digestive Disorders Foundation, 3 St Andrews Place, London NW1 4LB; www.digestivedisorders.org.uk
IBD Club	IBD Club, The Tower Building, 11 York Road, London SE1 7NX; www.ibdclub.org.uk

Use of nonsteroidal anti-inflammatory drugs

NSAIDs have been reported to exacerbate or lead to re-activation of pre-existing IBD. A prospective case-control study showed the risk of incident colitis with current and recent exposure to NSAIDs to be increased, with odds ratios of 2.96 and 2.51, respectively. The ability of NSAIDs to exacerbate pre-existing IBD may be related to inhibition of colonic prostaglandin synthesis. COX-2 expression in epithelial cells is increased in active disease, and may have a protective role. One *in vitro* study suggests the inhibition of prostanoid production by a highly selective COX-2 inhibitor is similar to that of a traditional nonselective NSAID. We advise patients with IBD to avoid NSAIDs whenever possible. The risks of COX-2 inhibitors exacerbating or re-activating IBD in clinical practice remains to be established.

Induction of remission

5-ASA agents, steroids, immunomodulatory therapy, biological therapy, antibiotics, nutritional therapy and heparin are used alone or in combination to induce remission in active IBD.

5-ASA agents

5-ASA agents are available orally, or as enema and suppositories. 5-ASA is the active component in the original sulfasalazine. The newer preparations consist of 5-ASA azo-linked to different carriers. The site of release/action generally determines the choice of oral agents. Newer agents are better tolerated than sulfasalazine (*Table 11.3*).

Table 11.3. Choice of 5-ASA agents

Oral formulation	Constituent	Site of release/action
Pentasa®	5-ASA	Duodenum to colon
Salofalk®	5-ASA	pH > 6, ileum, colon
Asacol®	5-ASA	pH > 7, distal ileum, colon
Sulfasalazine	5-ASA and sulfapyridine	Colon
Olsalazine	5-ASA dimer	Colon
Balsalazide	5-ASA, 4-aminobenzoyl and β-alanine	Colon

Steroids

Like 5-ASA agents, steroids are also available orally, or as enema and suppositories. Intravenous or oral steroids are used to treat moderate to severely active IBD. Topical steroids have been shown to be beneficial in distal colitis (*Table 11.4*).

Table 11.4. Choice of steroids

Steroids	Suggested regime	Problems
Prednisolone (oral)	40 mg for 1 week, 30 mg 1 week, 20 mg 4 weeks, thereafter decrease by 5 mg week^{-1}	Sleep and mood disturbance, Cushing's syndrome, narrow angle glaucoma, cataracts, osteoporosis
Budesonide (oral)	9 mg day^{-1}, decreasing by 3 mg	'Less' side-effects than standard steroids but 'greater' than placebo

Immunomodulatory therapy

Azathioprine and 6-mercaptopurine (6-MP) are effective treatment for inducing remission in chronic active IBD but the therapeutic effect takes up to 3 months. They have no role in acute severe disease due to the slow onset of action. Their main use has been in steroid sparing maintenance of remission (see *Table 11.5*).

Table 11.5. Immunomodulatory agents for inducing or maintaining remission

Immunomodulatory agents	Type of IBD	Suggested regime	Problems/side-effects
Azathioprine or 6-MP (used concomitantly with another drug initially)	CD (including perianal disease), UC	Oral azathioprine 2–3.0 mg kg day^{-1}, oral 6-MP 1–1.5 mg kg day^{-1}	Slow onset of action, intolerance, serious side-effects of pancreatitis, bone marrow suppression
Cyclosporin	UC, selected CD	4 mg kg day^{-1} i.v. with blood level monitoring, then change to oral 8 mg kg day^{-1}	Renal insufficiency, hypertrichosis, tremor, hypertension, headache, opportunistic infections
Methotrexate	CD	25 mg week^{-1} i.m. for 16 weeks, then change to 15 mg week^{-1} i.m.	Liver fibrosis, hypersensitivity pneumonitis, tetragenocity

IBD, inflammatory bowel disease; 6-MP, 6-mercaptopurine; CD, Crohn's disease; UC, ulcerative colitis.

Biological therapy

Infliximab, a chimeric IgG1 TNFα monoclonal antibody, has been shown to decrease morbidity and improve quality of life in CD. A placebo-controlled study showed a single infusion of 5 mg kg^{-1} has resulted in clinical improvement of 82% of patients and clinical remission in 48% of patients with chronic active CD at 4 weeks.

A course of three doses of infliximab given at 0, 2 and 6 weeks resulted in a ≥50% reduction in the number of draining fistulae in 68% of patients. Complete fistula closure was achieved in 55% of patients who received a dosage of 5 mg kg^{-1}. Median duration of closure time was 3 months.

As yet, there is no good evidence to support the use of infliximab in UC.

Antibiotics

Metronidazole and ciprofloxacin are the two commonly used antibiotics in mild to moderate CD or fistulating disease. The effect may be due to alteration of bacterial flora, and the antibiotics may also have innate immunomodulatory activity.

Nutritional therapy

Elemental diet when used as exclusive source of nutrition is effective in inducing remission of active CD. It is not useful for UC. Nutritional support via elemental feeding or parenteral nutrition is indicated for hospitalized IBD patients after 7 days if they are unable to maintain adequate caloric intake. Preoperative use of parenteral nutrition for severely malnourished patients, more commonly in CD, can improve outcome.

Heparin

Unfractionated heparin has been shown to be helpful in mild to moderate UC. The exact mechanism of action remains unclear.

Maintaining remission

5-ASA agents, immunomodulatory therapy and biological therapy are important in maintenance of remission in IBD.

Steroids

Steroids have no place in maintaining remission either for CD or UC and long-term use should be avoided.

5-ASA agents

The use of 5-ASA agents in maintenance therapy leads to a four- to fivefold reduction in relapses. The evidence for efficacy is stronger in UC than in CD. It is recommended that the patients on maintenance 5-ASA agents treatment have 6–12-monthly urea and creatinine checked. These agents are generally continued long term if tolerated.

Immunomodulatory therapy

Azathioprine and 6-MP are the most commonly used and effective immunosuppressants in CD and UC. About 10–15% of patients are intolerant due to side-effects such as nausea, vomiting, abdominal pain, worsening diarrhea, myalgia and arthralgia. Serious side-effects, such as pancreatitis and drug-related hepatitis, are not common. Bone marrow suppression requires regular blood count monitoring. Genetic polymorphisms of an enzyme, thiopurine methyltransferase (TPMT), give rise to a trimodal phenotypic expression of enzyme activity. Deficiency or low enzyme activity is associated with high risk of bone marrow suppression. Genotyping or assay for TPMT activity before starting thiopurine has been recommended, but the assays are not widely available. A suggested protocol for monitoring full blood count is 2-weekly for the first 3 months of treatment, and 2–3-monthly thereafter for as long as therapy is continued. The treatment is generally continued for 4 years. A trial of withdrawal can be considered after 4 years if the patients remain in remission.

Thiopurines are often started following successful induction of remission with cyclosporin and infliximab. Oral cyclosporin has been used following a successful response to intravenous cyclosporin in fulminant UC, but long-term use is not recommended. A recent study suggests methotrexate may be a useful maintenance therapy in CD (see *Table 11.5*).

Biological therapy

Repeated treatment of infliximab every 8 weeks in CD maintains the clinical benefit for 44 weeks, with a remission rate of 53%. Concurrent use of thiopurine may result in better clinical response.

Osteoporosis

Osteoporosis is an important cause of morbidity in IBD. This appears to be more common in CD and the pathogenesis probably involves disease inflammatory activity, plus contributory factors such as steroid use, calcium and vitamin D malabsorption. For prevention of osteoporosis, patients should be advised to have regular exercise, stop smoking, avoid excess alcohol and maintain adequate dietary calcium intake. For patients taking steroids, especially those requiring prolonged or multiple courses, consideration should be given to vitamin D supplementation or bisphosphonate.

Older patients are more at risk of osteoporosis and should have bone densitometry studies at presentation with IBD. If osteoporosis is diagnosed, treatment options include HRT (in postmenopausal women), bisphosphonate or calcitonin.

Cancer surveillance (see also Chapter 10)

Studies suggest that there is an increased risk of colon carcinoma in patients with CD as well as UC. This risk may be affected by duration and extent of disease, age of onset, presence of PSC and family history of colon cancer. The efficacy of current strategies of colonoscopic screening/surveillance for cancer in IBD remains an issue of debate. It is important to stress to the patients that colonoscopic surveillance does not prevent the development of cancer. There are also the inherent risks attached to the procedure. This needs to be discussed with individual patients given the wide publicity on the subject.

Crohn's disease

Induction of remission

5-ASA agents (see also section on Induction of remission under General management)

5-ASA agents are often prescribed for induction of remission. The data on efficacy is less impressive when compared to those in UC. The choice of 5-ASA depends on the location of the disease. Pentasa®, Salofalk® and Asacol® are all released in small and large bowel. For disease confined to the colon, sulfasalazine and olsalazine, which are hydrolyzed by colonic bacteria are more appropriate. Sulfasalazine has been found to be helpful in ileocolonic or colonic disease.

Antibiotics

Antibiotics are an option in management of mild to moderate active CD, and treatment of perianal disease (see *Table 11.6*).

Table 11.6. Choice of antibiotics in Crohn's disease

Indications	Suggested regime	Problems
Mild to moderate ileocolitis or colitis, perianal disease	Metronidazole 10–20 mg kg^{-1} day^{-1}, for 4–6 months	Anorexia, nausea/vomiting, disulfiram like effect, prolonged use is associated with peripheral neuropathy.
As above	Ciprofloxacin 1 g daily, alone or with above	Nausea/vomiting, rash, pseudomembranous colitis

Steroids (see also section on Induction of remission under General management)

For moderate to severe symptoms of CD, steroids are the most effective treatment. Unfortunately, many patients treated acutely with steroids may become steroid dependent. The risk factors for this include smoking and colonic disease. Budesonide may be helpful in patients with mildly active ileal/ileocecal disease. Its benefit in patients with more severe disease is disappointing.

Immunomodulatory therapy (see *Table 11.5*)

Azathioprine and 6-MP are effective treatments for chronic active CD. The slow onset of action necessitates concurrent short-term use of steroids.

Methotrexate given intramuscularly is effective in inducing remission for CD and may be suitable for the patients intolerant to thiopurines.

Biological therapy

Infliximab decreases morbidity and improves quality of life in CD. It is effective in chronic active CD and fistulating CD (see *Table 11.7*).

Table 11.7. Use of infliximab in Crohn's disease (CD)

Indications	Suggested regime	Problems
Refractory chronic active CD	Induction – 5 mg kg^{-1} single infusion	Infusion reactions, delayed hypersensitivity reactions, HACA, drug-induced lupus
	Maintenance – repeat infusion of 10 mg kg^{-1} every 8 weeks	
Fistulating CD	5 mg kg^{-1} single infusion, repeated at 2 and 6 weeks	As above

HACA, human antichimeric antibody

Nutritional therapy – enteral nutrition (see also Chapter 16)

Elemental diet when used as an exclusive source of nutrition can induce remission of active CD, but it is probably less effective than steroids. The long-term benefit is less than satisfactory, with 70% relapse of symptoms with re-introduction of regular food. The cost is considerable and poor palatability sometimes necessitates administration via a nasogastric tube.

Assessment as inpatients

Patients with severe/fulminant disease presentation will require hospitalization and parenteral steroids. A helpful working definition (practice guideline, American College of Gastroenterology) of severe/fulminant disease is persistence of symptoms despite introduction of steroids as outpatients, or individuals presenting with high fever, persistent vomiting, evidence of intestinal obstruction, rebound tenderness, cachexia or evidence of an abscess.

Surgical referral may be warranted for the patients who have severe intractable/fulminant disease requiring hospitalization and parenteral steroids.

Surgical assessment is also helpful for the following:

- Recurrent small bowel or large bowel obstruction (resection or stricturoplasty)
- Abscess (perianal or intra-abdominal)
- Fistula (perianal, rectovaginal or small bowel)
- Entero-enteric fistulas are often asymptomatic and may respond to medical therapy

Maintaining remission

5-ASA agents and steroids

5-ASA agents have not generally been shown to be effective in maintenance treatment although mesalazine may be effective as maintenance therapy if it induced the remission. Steroids have no place as long-term maintenance therapy.

Immunomodulatory therapy

Azathioprine and 6-MP are an effective steroid-sparing maintenance therapy in chronic active disease and for those patients who suffer from frequent relapses.

A placebo-controlled withdrawal study showed methotrexate 15 mg week^{-1} i.m. for 40 weeks to be an effective maintenance agent following the remission induction by a course of i.m. methotrexate. Sixty-five per cent of methotrexate-treated patients remained in remission compared to 39% for those receiving placebo injection. Liver toxicity is not a problem for cumulative doses of up to 5 g. Folic acid supplementation is helpful for side-effects and hematological toxicity.

Mycophenolate at 15 mg kg^{-1} day^{-1} given orally may be an option for those patients intolerant of thiopurines and/or methotrexate. Its place in routine practice remains to be established.

Biological agents

Early data from the ACCENT-I trial (A Crohn's Disease Clinical Trial Evaluating Infliximab in a new Long-term Treatment Regimen) suggests that maintenance therapy with repeated infliximab infusion every 8 weeks improves clinical response and remission rate when compared to single-dose treatment (Hanauer *et al.*, 2001). Retreatment appears to prolong remissions in the patients with moderate to severe CD.

Perianal disease

The use of metronidazole alone or in combination with ciprofloxacin is effective in nonsuppurative perianal disease. Thiopurine use may result in long-term improvement. Intravenous infliximab given in a series of three doses was shown to have clear benefits in refractory Crohn's fistulae. Perianal or perirectal abscesses require surgical drainage.

Postsurgical patients

Endoscopic studies suggest the presence of endoscopic recurrence in up to 70% of patients within 1 year of surgery, although symptomatic recurrence is less frequent and often delayed. The risk of postoperative recurrence is greater with longer duration of disease, steroid intake during the 6 months preceding surgery, older age and smoking.

There is some evidence to support postoperative use of Pentasa® (> 3 g day^{-1}), antibiotics or thiopurines to maintain remission.

Smoking

Smoking cigarettes may influence the course of disease. Studies suggest heavy smokers required more operations and were more likely to have fistulae and abscesses, and smoking increases the risk of small bowel CD and relapsing disease. Smoking has a negative impact on the course of CD, with increased likelihood of disease recurrence. Patients should be advised to stop smoking.

Dietary alteration

A low residue diet will help decrease obstructive symptoms in the patients with inflammatory narrowing of small intestine or subacute obstruction. Patients with fibrotic narrowing, however, will require stricture resection or stricturoplasty.

Continuing diarrhea symptoms at follow-up

If patients complain of ongoing diarrhea symptoms, despite an apparent clinical picture of clinical remission, one needs to consider IBS/functional bowel symptoms that often coexist with IBD. In postsurgical patients, the differential diagnosis also includes bile salt malabsorption and bacterial overgrowth. Coexisting celiac disease is rare but this is usually diagnosed late. Lastly, the possibility of active or recurrent CD needing further investigations should be borne in mind (*Table 11.8*).

Table 11.8. Investigations and management for continuing diarrhea symptoms

Problems	Tests		Treatment
Bile salt malabsorption	^{75}SeHCAT (7-day retention) or empirical cholestyramine therapy	Especially if previous terminal ileal resection/ right hemicolectomy	Cholestyramine
Bacterial overgrowth	Lactulose hydrogen breath test	As above	Rotating antibiotics
Discrepancy between clinical symptoms and structural/anatomic studies	^{99m}Tc HMPAO scan	Labeled white cell scan helps discriminate areas with inflammatory activity	

HMPAO, hexamethyl propylenamine oxine

Vitamin B$_{12}$ deficiency

Patients with limited ileal resection (< 100 cm) with or without right hemi-colectomy are at risk of vitamin B$_{12}$ malabsorption. Such patients require intra-muscular supplementation every 2–3 months for life.

Ulcerative colitis

Induction of remission

5-ASA agents

In mild to moderate disease, both oral and topical 5-ASA agents are effective initial treatment. They induce complete remission in at least 50% of the cases. The choices include pentasa, sulfasalazine, olsalazine or balsalazide, the latter two preferred in distal disease. The addition of oral steroids increases successful remission rate to near 90%. The latter should be started in moderate to severely active disease. The evidence remains inconclusive regarding whether combined topical and oral 5-ASA agents are more effective than either agent alone.

Steroids

As in CD, steroids are effective therapy to induce remission for mild to severe UC.

Heparin

Uncontrolled studies showed 4–6 weeks of unfractionated heparin in steroid-resistant UC result in clinical remission of over 70%. The effect may be due to immunomodulatory and anti-inflammatory rather than anticoagulant prop-erties. This is often prescribed as adjunctive treatment for inpatients, but the use for prolonged periods as outpatients may be logistically difficult.

Assessment as inpatients

Patients who have severe disease as evidenced by diarrhea > 10 times per day, abdominal distention and tenderness, fever, tachycardia, anemia and leucocytosis will require hospitalization and parenteral steroids. In the absence of objective improvement in 5–7 days, i.v. cyclosporin 4 mg kg^{-1} day^{-1} is used as rescue therapy for acute severe UC as an alternative to surgery. Long-term use of this nephrotoxic drug is not recommended. CRP > 45 at day 4 indicates severe disease and is useful clinically in the decision to start cyclosporin or consider surgery.

Failure to respond or worsening symptoms are indications for surgery. Other indications for surgery include toxic megacolon, massive hemorrhage or obstruction resulting from stricture.

Maintaining remission

5-ASA agents

Oral or rectal 5-ASA agents have been shown to be effective maintenance therapy in UC. They decrease the annual relapse rate from 70–80% with placebo to 20–30%. Long-term use of rectal formulations may be hampered by patient compliance.

Immunomodulatory agents

Thiopurines are beneficial for those patients who are steroid dependent or suffer from frequent relapses.

For those patients with severe fulminant colitis who improve on i.v. cyclosporin, the use of oral thiopurine improves long-term outcome.

Box 11.2	Summary of issues to consider at follow-up clinic

- Education
- Lifestyle modifications – smoking, diet, avoiding nonsteroidal anti-inflammatory drugs
- Optimize induction treatment (new patients or flare up)
- Admit acutely ill patients for further assessment if needed
- Optimize maintenance therapy for remission
- Prevention of complications – osteoporosis, B$_{12}$ injection
- Investigations/therapy for continuing diarrhea
- Cancer surveillance

Further reading

Calkins, B.M. (1989) A meta-analysis of the role of smoking in inflammatory bowel disease. *Dig. Dis. Sci.* **34**: 1841–1854.

Camma, C., Giunta, M., Toselli, M. and Cottone, M. (1997) Mesalamine in the maintenance treatment of Crohn's disease: a meta-analysis adjusted for confounding. *Gastroenterology* **113**: 1465–1473.

Forbes, A. (2001) *Inflammatory Bowel Disease: A Clinician's Guide.* 2nd edition. Oxford University Press, Oxford.

Franceschi, S., Panza, E., La Vecchia, C., Parazzini, F., Decarli, A., Bianchi Porro, G. (1987) Nonspecific inflammatory disease and smoking. *Am. J. Epidemiol.* **125**: 445–452.

Hanauer, S.B., Lichtenstein, G.R., Clumbel, J.F., *et al.* (2001) Maintenance infliximab (Remicade) is safe, effective and steroid sparing in Crohn's disease: preliminary results from ACCENT I Trial. *Gastroenterology* **120** (Suppl. I): A21.

Orholm, M., Munkholm, P., Lamgholz, E., Nielsen, O.H., Sorensen, I.A. and Binder, V. (1991) Familial occurrence of inflammatory bowel disease. *N. Eng. J. Med.* **324**: 84–88.

Rampton, D. (2000) *Inflammatory Bowel Disease: Clinical Diagnosis and Management.* 1st edition. Blackwell Science, Oxford.

Satsangi, J., Jewell, D.P., Rosenberg, W.M.C. and Bell, J.I. (1994) Genetics of inflammatory bowel disease. *Gut* **35**: 696–700.

Stotland, B.R., Stein, R.B. and Lichtenstein, G.R. (2000) Advances in inflammatory bowel disease. Med. *Clin. North Am.* **84**: 1107–1124.

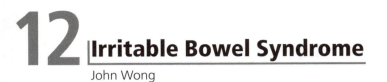

12 Irritable Bowel Syndrome

John Wong

Introduction

IBS has been defined as a functional bowel disorder in which abdominal pain is associated with defecation or a change of bowel habit, with features of disordered defecation and distention. The criteria for diagnosis have evolved from the Manning criteria in 1978 to the Rome I criteria in 1988. The latter were revised to Rome II criteria in 1998 (*Box 12.1*; Thompson *et al.*, 2000).

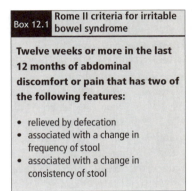

Box 12.1	Rome II criteria for irritable bowel syndrome

Twelve weeks or more in the last 12 months of abdominal discomfort or pain that has two of the following features:

- relieved by defecation
- associated with a change in frequency of stool
- associated with a change in consistency of stool

In clinical as well as research practice, IBS is classified into diarrhea- or constipation-predominant IBS, or alternate constipation/diarrhea IBS. These symptomatic criteria are useful clinically and classification facilitates research and allows comparability of studies of drug treatment.

Epidemiology

IBS is the most common functional bowel disorder, affecting 9–12% of the population. It is twice as common in women than in men, affecting approximately 5% of men and 13% of women in the UK. Patients with IBS symptoms form 20–50% of gastroenterology referrals. A study of IBS in general practice showed a prevalence of 30% among the patients presenting with a GI complaint. On average, GPs see one new case and seven repeat visits a week.

Pathophysiology

IBS is considered a biopsychosocial disorder as a consequence of psychosocial factors, altered motility and transit, and increased sensitivity of the intestine and colon.

Autonomic dysfunction has been described in IBS, with decreased vagal tone in patients with constipation and increased sympathetic activity when diarrhea predominates. Colonic transit and propagated contractions are increased in diarrhea-predominant IBS. More recent interest has been centered on altered sensation of the intestine and colon, as well as the central nervous system processing of afferent information. The latter may ultimately explain the association between IBS and mood and psychosocial stressors, as well as disease beliefs and expectations.

Infectious diarrhea with *Campylobacter*, *Shigella* and *Salmonella* has been associated with persistent bowel dysfunction in 25% of patients. The predisposing factors include a physically more severe dysenteric episode, life event, stress and anxiety preceding the acute illness. An episode of culture positive bacterial gastroenteritis is a strong predictor of new-onset IBS (relative risk 11.9).

Contributory factors to irritable bowel syndrome symptoms

Carbohydrate intolerance plays a role in symptoms for some IBS patients, and these include lactose and fructose intolerance. The prevalence of lactose intolerance varies between ethnic groups and the symptoms are dependent on total carbohydrate load. Impaired digestion probably leads to excess gas formation and consequent bloating symptoms, and osmotically active metabolites cause diarrhea. Some patients are also sensitive to sorbitol and mannitol, which are used as artificial sweeteners in dietetic food.

About 10% of diarrhea-predominant IBS patients have evidence of bile salt malabsorption. A clinical diagnosis is often made following a positive response to a trial of cholestyramine. This can be confirmed with the finding of decreased body retention of ^{75}SeHCAT, a radioactive analog of cholyltaurine.

Depression and anxiety are the most common comorbid affective disorders in IBS.

Psychological symptoms, such as somatization, anxiety, hostility, phobia and paranoia, are more common in patients with IBS. Psychosocial factors can modulate the experience of somatic symptoms and contribute to abnormal illness behavior, increased physician consultations and reduced coping capability.

Diagnosis and management approach (see *Figure 12.1*)

IBS is the most common GI condition in general practice but less than a third of patients are referred to specialists. The diagnosis is often made in the primary care setting (*Box 12.2*).

Non-GI symptoms such as nocturia, frequency and urgency of micturition, incomplete bladder emptying, back pain, unpleasant taste in the mouth, a constant feeling of tiredness and dyspareunia are more

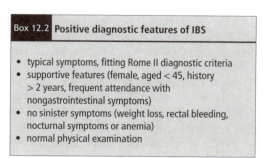

Box 12.2 **Positive diagnostic features of IBS**

- typical symptoms, fitting Rome II diagnostic criteria
- supportive features (female, aged < 45, history > 2 years, frequent attendance with nongastrointestinal symptoms)
- no sinister symptoms (weight loss, rectal bleeding, nocturnal symptoms or anemia)
- normal physical examination

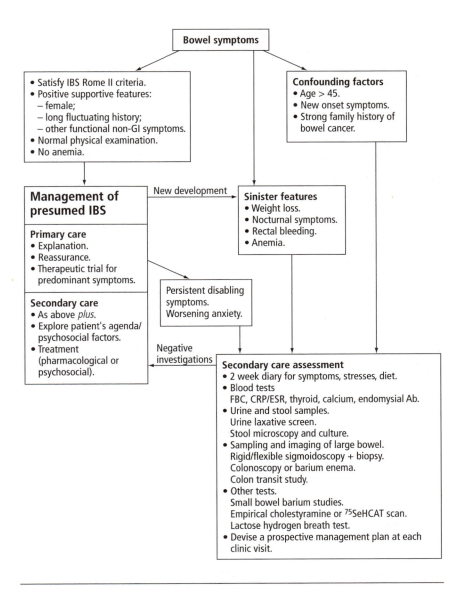

Figure 12.1. A management approach to irritable bowel syndrome

common in IBS patients than in control subjects. These symptoms could serve to support the diagnosis of IBS.

Patients referred to secondary care have often been filtered and are more likely to have atypical features suggesting organic pathology, or those regarded as 'difficult to manage' by the GP. Other features of patients seen in secondary care are:

- Patients that tend not to recognize psychological factors in illness, and have often failed to be reassured after some 'baseline' blood tests and possibly radiological or endoscopy examination. They remain concerned that something is still amiss, justified by their persistent symptoms
- Patients that have already been tried on empirical medications, such as smooth muscle relaxants, or that self-medicate with over-the-counter medicine and/or dietary manipulation
- A significant number of patients that are very conversant with the diagnosis from the knowledge gained from friends, relatives or through the internet

These patients often have waited a long time for a clinic appointment as their referrals tend to be graded as routine in the absence of alarm features and may be frustrated.

Bearing in mind the above considerations, consultations for IBS patients in the secondary care setting often require an ample amount of time, patience and empathy. Establishing an effective physician–patient relationship and sizing up the patients' agenda are crucial to effective management of patients.

IBS symptoms often fluctuate over time, resulting in repeated referrals and repetitive investigations. Any perception of unsatisfactory interaction with the healthcare system by the patients, often involving prolonged wait for unpleasant tests, may be contributory to distress and continued healthcare-seeking behavior. It is important not to dismiss patients with a previous diagnosis of IBS, paying particular attention to atypical features such as rectal bleeding or anemia. A thorough physical examination and a limited series of initial investigations are needed to exclude organic structural, metabolic or infectious diseases.

Differential diagnosis and investigations

These include lactose intolerance, celiac disease, diverticular disease, drug-induced diarrhea or constipation, biliary tract disease, laxative abuse, parasitic disease, microscopic (collagenous) colitis and early inflammatory bowel disease.

Diagnostic tests should be 'targeted' with the above differential diagnosis in mind, and the number of 'screening' blood tests or radiological imaging limited (see *Table 12.1*).

Exploration of patient's agenda/psychosocial factors

The patient may have been symptomatic for years but was referred now because of a triggering event or perception that their symptoms are getting worse. Fear of cancer is common in IBS patients, with one study showing 46% prevalence as compared to 30% in controls with organic disease. The fear may be justifiable from a strong family history of colon carcinoma. Other factors influencing health-seeking behavior include severity and duration of abdominal pain symptoms, rather than psychological factors. Psychiatric features cannot be used reliably to distinguish functional from organic disease.

Table 12.1. Investigations for presumed IBS

Problems	Tests	Details	
New onset change in bowel habit age > 45, strong family history of colon cancer	Colonoscopy or barium enema	Large bowel evaluation	Rule out colon cancer
Diarrhea-predominant symptoms	Blood tests	Thyroid function, CRP, ESR, endomysial antibody	Exclude hyperthyroidism, inflammatory bowel disease, celiac disease
	Stool	Microscopy and culture	Rule out parasitic infection
	Endoscopy	Rigid or flexible sigmoidoscopy and random biopsies	Inflammatory bowel disease or microscopic colitis
	Urine	Laxative screen	Laxative abuse
	^{75}SeHCAT or empirical cholestyramine	7-day retention	Bile salt malabsorption
	Breath test	Lactose hydrogen	Lactose intolerance in those consuming >280 ml milk or diary products
	Barium studies	Small bowel studies	Crohn's disease
Constipation-predominant symptoms	Bloods	Thyroid function, calcium level	Hypothyroidism, hypercalcemia
	Radiology	Colon transit study	Large bowel dysmotility

CRP, C-reactive protein; ESR, erythrocyte sedimentation rate

Explanation/reassurance

A satisfactory explanation of the diagnosis, and the idea of brain–gut axis inter-action for IBS symptoms, help to reassure the patients. A 2-week diary to include symptoms, stresses and diet may be helpful in identifying aggravating factors and could form the basis of management discussion. One study suggests that only 26% of patients with IBS felt entirely better about their symptoms after their visit to the GP. This may be a reflection of the complexity of these patients or inadequate consultation time for detailed explanation. Many clinical studies of IBS treatment show a high placebo-response rate, which may persist during 1 year of treatment. While this demonstrates the therapeutic potential of a placebo, it also illustrates that the comprehensive follow-up practiced in clinical studies (such as weekly telephone contact) serves as psychological reassurance for many patients, which can be therapeutic in its own right. A 'negotiated' regular outpatient follow-up arrangement may be suitable for some patients in place of medications and probably avoids their rapid return as a new referral.

Treatment (pharmacological or psychological)

There is no proven specific treatment for the entire IBS symptom complex, although clinical studies support the efficacy of some medications for global improvement or individual symptoms.

A therapeutic trial (if not already initiated by the GP) for the predominant symptoms is worthwhile. One of the medications in a therapeutic class may be more effective in an individual, and sequential trials of different drugs in the same group may be helpful. This benefit may be due to repetitive placebo effects. It helps to plan ahead for the next clinic visit and provide the patients with a prospective management plan.

Constipation-predominant irritable bowel syndrome

Diet

Fiber increases colonic transit in constipation-predominant IBS. There are few randomized or mechanistic studies of fiber in IBS. Although clinical studies of bulking agents thus far do not shown efficacy on specific symptoms such as bowel frequency and abdominal pain, some suggest global improvement in symptoms. Consumption of 20–30 g day^{-1} fiber leads to significant improvement in constipation.

Unfortunately, a high-fiber diet often exacerbates the symptom of bloating. If bloating is a prominent feature, patients are advised to avoid dietary beans, cabbage and other food containing fermentable carbohydrates. A practicable exclusion rather than a formal elimination diet are easier to comply with and may be helpful for some patients.

Lactulose and synthetic fiber can be prescribed for use on a regular basis; the latter may be better tolerated than natural fiber. The use of stimulant laxatives should be restricted to the short term or as required basis wherever possible.

Antispasmodics

Antispasmodics are commonly prescribed in IBS, and studies showed them to be effective in patients whose predominant symptom is abdominal pain. The commonly used dicycloverine (Merbentyl®) and hyoscine (Buscopan®) are anticholinergic and may be associated with antimuscarinic side-effects. Alverine (Spasmonal®), mebeverine (Colofac®) or peppermint oil (Colpermin®) have more direct inhibitory effect on intestinal smooth muscle.

Psychotropic treatment

A meta-analysis of antidepressants in functional GI disorders (including 11 reports of IBS patients) suggest there was an eightfold benefit for pain and 4.4-fold benefit for global or symptomatic improvement compared with control therapy. Antidepressants have neuromodulatory and analgesic effects, and this may benefit IBS patients independent of their psychotropic properties. The rationale of this needs to be explained to the patients who may be skeptical of taking an antidepressant. They need to be taken continually for 4–6 weeks before a therapeutic effect can be excluded. The choice of antidepressant agent depends on the predominant bowel symptoms, any sleep disturbance or anxiety disorders.

Previous studies mostly used tricyclic agents, which are associated with constipation. These appear more beneficial in those with abdominal pain and diarrhea (see below). More recently, SSRIs such as paroxetine and citalopram have been used although there are, as yet, no published randomized controlled studies confirming their efficacy. They may induce diarrhea and this could be advantageous for constipation-predominant IBS.

An alternative in patients with pain symptoms in IBS is to try active psychotherapeutic therapy such as cognitive behavioral therapy (CBT) and dynamic or interpersonal therapy. The more passive treatment options include relaxation therapy and hypnotherapy. These treatments are time consuming and they are not universally available. A multicenter UK study found that psychotherapy and an SSRI (paroxetine) improve health-related quality of life and the treatment costs are favorable compared to 'treatment as usual'. More randomized studies are needed to identify the subgroup of patients who will benefit from each individual approach.

Serotonin modulators

Serotonin (5HT) is involved in the sensory and motor functions of the gut, and modifies motility and secretion in the gut via a number of receptors (types 3 and 4).

The activation of 5HT4 can promote peristalsis and increase fluid release into the gut. In a large multicenter study, Tegaserod (a partial 5HT4 agonist) produced improvement in subjective global relief of symptoms in female patients with constipation-predominant IBS. There was also improvement in daily bloating score, and three bowel-related assessments including stool frequency, consistency and straining. This drug is awaiting licensing approval in the USA.

Diarrhea-predominant irritable bowel syndrome

Diet

Lactose intolerance occurs in about 10% of patients with IBS. However, patients are unlikely to benefit from lactose restriction unless their daily consumption of lactose exceeds a 0.5 pint (280 ml) of milk equivalent.

Patients are encouraged to keep a detailed food diary and experiment with a practicable exclusion diet, focusing on those commonly reporting intolerance including wheat, dairy products (cheese, yogurt and milk), coffee, potatoes, corn, onions, beef, oats and white wine. The therapeutic effect of fiber in diarrhea symptoms remains uncertain.

True food allergy is rare and should only be diagnosed with objective history or signs of urticaria, bronchospasm, angio-edema or rash. These patients should be referred to immunologists.

Loperamide

Diarrhea-predominant IBS is associated with acceleration of small bowel and proximal colonic transit and respond to opioids. Loperamide is a synthetic opioid, which works by decreasing intestinal transit, enhancing intestinal water and ion absorption and increases anal sphincter tone at rest. It improves symptoms of diarrhea, urgency and fecal soiling. The dose requirement should be titrated to avoid constipation. It can be used prophylactically in anticipation of precipitating factors for bowel symptoms, for instance stressful events including social encounters.

Codeine phosphate is similarly effective but may cause sedation.

Cholestyramine

A therapeutic trial of cholestyramine can be given for suspected cases of bile salt malabsorption in IBS. Bile acid sequestrant therapy has been shown to be helpful where antidiarrheal drugs have failed in patients with chronic diarrhea/IBS. Successful response depends on 7-day [75]SeHCAT retention being < 5%. If cholestyramine is not tolerated in confirmed bile acid malabsorption, cholestipol hydrochloride can be tried instead.

Antispasmodics – see Constipation-predominant IBS above

Psychotropic treatment

Low-dose tricyclics (e.g. 10–25 mg amitriptyline) are helpful for diarrhea and pain symptoms in IBS. The antimuscarinic side-effect is probably responsible for improvement of diarrhea symptoms. The drug is taken at night and some benefit may be a result of better sleep. Trazodone (tricyclic-related) has fewer anti-muscarinic effect and is helpful if insomnia is a significant problem.

Predominance of diarrhea and pain, an association with overt psychiatric symptoms, or intermittent pain exacerbated by stress were shown to be predictive factors for a favorable response for psychotherapy.

Serotonin modulator

The antagonism of 5HT3 receptors increases the thresholds for sensation and discomfort during distention of rectum, increases colonic compliance, slows colonic transit and improves stool consistency. Alosetron, a selective 5HT3 antagonist, was shown to improve pain, urgency and stool frequency in female patients with alternating and diarrhea-predominant IBS. Unfortunately, adverse events of acute ischemic colitis occur in 0.1–1% of patients. It was withdrawn from the market in the USA in November 2000.

Another promising 5HT3 antagonist, cilansetron, is currently undergoing clinical studies. One recent study in nonconstipated IBS patients showed efficacy in adequate relief of symptoms for both male and female patients. It also showed improvement of abdominal pain, stool frequency and consistency.

Helpful contact

Penny Nunn, IBS network, Northern General Hospital, Sheffield S5 7AU, UK; www.ibsnetwork.org.uk

Further reading

Akehurst, R. and Kaltenthaler, E. (2001) Treatment of irritable bowel syndrome: a review of randomised controlled trials. *Gut* **48**: 272–282.

Camilleri, M. (2001) Management of the irritable bowel syndrome. *Gastroenterology* **120**: 652–668.

Jailwala, J., Imperiale, T.F. and Kroenke, K. (2000) Pharmacologic treatment of the irritable bowel syndrome: a systematic review of randomised controlled trials. *Ann. Intern. Med.* **133**: 136–147.

Jones, J., Boorman, J., Cann, P., *et al*. (2000) British Society of Gastroenterology guidelines for the management of the irritable bowel syndrome. *Gut* **47** (Suppl II): ii1–19.

Thompson, W.G., Longstreth, G.F., Drossman, D.A., *et al.* (1999) Functional bowel disorders and functional abdominal pain. *Gut* **45**: II43–II47.

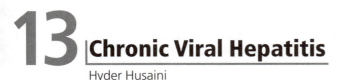

Chronic Viral Hepatitis

Hyder Husaini

Introduction

Chronic viral hepatitis is the main worldwide cause for chronic liver disease, cirrhosis and hepatocellular cancer. Chronic viral hepatitis can be defined as a hepatocellular inflammation or necrosis for more than 6 months as a result of a viral infection. Hepatitis B (HBV) with or without hepatitis D, and hepatitis C (HCV) can lead to persistent infection and chronic hepatitis. Hepatitis A and E are self-limiting viral infections that do not lead to chronic infection. Recent studies suggest that the hepatitis G virus may cause mild acute hepatitis but does not cause clinically significant chronic disease. This chapter discusses the management of chronic viral hepatitis in the outpatient clinic.

Epidemiology and natural history of chronic viral hepatitis

Chronic hepatitis B

More than 300 million people worldwide are infected by HBV, which is transmitted parentally. In Western communities, the commonest risk factors for transmission are intravenous drug abuse, unprotected sex, hemodialysis and occupational 'needle-stick injury'. Perinatal vertical transmission is the predominant mode of transmission in high HBV-prevalence areas with maternal transmission rates of 90% if the mother is hepatitis B e antigen (HBeAg) positive.

Natural history

Chronic HBV occurs in less than 1% of immunocompetent adults with a rate of clearance of hepatitis B surface antigen (HBsAg) of approximately 0.5% per year. The chances of developing chronic disease is greatest in infants infected at birth by vertical maternal transmission, men and those experiencing an asymptomatic or mild icteric illness or silent infection.

The prognosis of chronic HBV is variable. In patients with HBV from endemic areas, the prognosis is poorer than in Western patients who acquired HBV in adult life. Thus, the lifetime risk for HBV-related death in Chinese males is 50% and 15% for women. In contrast, in western HBsAg-positive blood donors, the majority remains asymptomatic with a very low risk of cirrhosis or hepatocellular carcinoma (HCC). For patients with compensated HBV cirrhosis, the 5-year survival is 80%, although for decompensated cirrhosis may be as low as 14%.

Factors affecting prognosis with chronic hepatitis B

The duration of HBV replication before clearance of the virus is the major factor in determining poorer prognosis as a result of a longer duration of necroinflammation. Other factors that adversely affect prognosis of chronic HBV infection include hepatitis D superinfection. The role of alcohol as a cofactor in acceleration of chronic HBV is uncertain and HCV coinfection seems to promote HBeAg seroconversion.

Chronic hepatitis C

HCV is an RNA flavivirus, first identified in 1989. The estimated prevalence of HCV infection in the UK varies between 200 000 and 400 000. The World Health Organization estimates that there are 170 million infected patients worldwide. Up to 85% of HCV-infected patients will progress to chronic liver disease.

Parental transmission of HCV is the major transmission route with between 50% and 100% of intravenous drug abusers, and 60–80% of hemophiliacs prior to blood product screening in 1991, being anti-HCV antibody positive. The risk factors are shown in *Figure 13.1*. Note that up to 25% have no apparent risk factors. Needle-stick injuries carry a low risk of transmission (1.8% estimated by the Center for Disease Control, USA, in 1997) with a low rate of seroconversion. Sexual transmission and vertical transmission also appear to be rare, unless patients are coinfected with HIV.

Genotype

There are six distinct genetic types of HCV, genotype 1 accounting for 40% of cases in the UK. The majority of the remaining cases are genotypes 2 and 3. Genotype may influence the rate of progression of disease; genotype 1 is found in those patients with more advanced disease and responds less well to antiviral therapy.

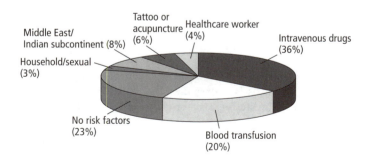

Figure 13.1. Route of acquisition of viral hepatitis C. Data from Watson *et al. Gut* 1996; 38: 269–276.

Natural history

Less than 10% of patients experience acute hepatitis; asymptomatic infection generally occurs. However, up to 85% of those infected with HCV will go onto chronic infection being both antibody positive to HCV and positive for serum HCV RNA.

Chronic HCV infection is a slowly progressive disease with median time to cirrhosis of 30 years (range 13–42 years). Approximately 20–30% with chronic HCV will develop cirrhosis by 20 years, although, in contrast, 30% will not progress to cirrhosis for up to 50 years postinfection. Thus the rate of disease progression is variable with rapid progression more likely if infection is acquired over the age of 40, in males and if the patient drinks more than 50 g of alcohol a day. Coinfection with HBV or HIV increases the rate of disease progression. Transfusion-acquired HCV may also lead to more rapidly progressive disease.

In patients with established cirrhosis, the prognosis is reasonable with over 90% of patients surviving 5 years after the diagnosis of cirrhosis and a 5-year risk of developing hepatocellular carcinoma of 7%. Unfortunately, within 5 years of diagnosis, 18% of patients with cirrhosis may develop decompensated liver disease. The 5-year mortality rate in patients with decompensated HCV cirrhosis is 50%.

Diagnosis of chronic viral hepatitis

Chronic hepatitis B

Hepatitis B surface antigen

HBsAg is the major diagnostic criteria for HBV infection. In patients who recover from acute HBV, HBsAg is usually undetectable 6 months postacute illness. Chronic infection with HBV is defined as persistence of HBsAg for more than 6 months.

The disappearance of HBsAg is followed by the appearance of hepatitis B surface antibody (anti-HBs), although both HBsAg and anti-HBs can coexist in a quarter of HBsAg-positive individuals. In these patients, anti-HBs is unable to neutralize the circulating virions, thus these patients should be treated as chronic HBV.

Hepatitis B core antigen and antibody

Hepatitis B core antigen (HBcAg) is an intracellular antigen that is expressed in infected hepatocytes but not detectable in serum. Antibody to HBcAg (anti-HBc) can be detected throughout the course of HBV infection.

High titers of IgM anti-HBc are indicative of acute HBV infection, although lower titers can remain detectable up to 2 years after the acute infection. During exacerbations of chronic HBV, the titer of IgM anti-HBc may increase. IgG anti-HBc is indicative of past infection with HBV and is present in chronic HBV.

Hepatitis B e antigen and antibody

HBeAg is generally considered a marker of HBV replication and is usually associated with the detection of HBV DNA in serum. The seroconversion of HBeAg to antibody to HBeAg (anti-HBe) occurs early in patients with acute infection but HBeAg seroconversion may be delayed for years to decades in patients with chronic HBV infection.

Hepatitis B DNA

Three types of assays for HBV DNA in serum have been developed with differing sensitivities. The branched DNA (bDNA) and hybridization assays have a lower limit sensitivity of 100 000 to 1 million viral copies per ml. However, polymerase chain reaction (PCR) assays can detect as little as 50–1000 viral copies per ml. In patients with chronic HBV infection, HBeAg seroconversion is usually accompanied by the disappearance of HBV DNA in serum as detected by hybridization or bDNA assays, although PCR assays will remain positive except in patients who have HBsAg seroconversion.

Chronic hepatitis C

Hepatitis C antibody testing

The third-generation ELISA test using antigens, NS3, NS4 and NS5 regions from the HCV nucleocapsid have a sensitivity of 97% with seroconversion by 2–3 weeks after infection. False-positive ELISA tests can occur. Thus in patients who are a very low risk of HCV infection, a positive HCV ELISA is confirmed using a third-generation recombinant immunoblot assay (RIBA) for four HCV antigens (C22, C33, C100-3 and NS 5). A positive RIBA test (two or more antigens positive) correlates well with positive HCV RNA detection and allows for earlier detection of HCV infection in acute cases.

Hepatitis C RNA assay

PCR for HCV RNA detection using primers from the highly conserved 5′ noncoding region is now the gold standard for confirmation of HCV infection. Commercial assays have a sensitivity of between 500 and 1000 viral copies per ml.
Qualitative HCV PCR should be used to confirm:

- viremia prior to antiviral therapy
- lack of viremia postantiviral therapy
- indeterminate RIBA results
- acute infection
- infection in immunosuppressed patients

PCR for serum HCV RNA is mandatory before commencing antiviral treatment. HCV antibody testing may be negative in immunosuppressed patients suspected of HCV infection or those who are recently infected, thus PCR testing for serum

HCV can be used to confirm the diagnosis. Since 10–15% of patients spontaneously clear HCV infection, some patients will be HCV antibody positive but PCR negative for serum HCV RNA. These patients have repeat HCV PCR 6 months later to confirm viral clearance.

Outpatient management

In our practice, most of the HCV referrals come from the drug rehabilitation team. These patients have had, or are concurrently being treated, for substance abuse. We therefore have a joint clinic with a member of the rehabilitation team who has been trained in the management of chronic HCV. Patient compliance with this joint approach is very good and the success rate for HCV treatment has improved. The addition of a specialist nurse to the team is invaluable for education of the patient, follow-up in the community and outpatient follow-up whilst on treatment. All patients who require interferon treatment are admitted for a morning to a short-stay ward to obtain training on the administration of interferon and to have their first dose of interferon. All patients now receive written information about HCV and both GP and patient receive information sheets with regard to combination treatment with interferon and ribavirin. Chronic HBV is an infrequent problem in our practice and is treated in a separate hepatology clinic.

Preconsultation

In patients referred with HBV or HCV, we normally request LFTs and hepatitis virology. For patients who are HBsAg positive, hepatitis e antigen/antibody status is of use to determine whether an active viral replication is likely. For patients with positive hepatitis C antibody by ELISA and/or RIBA, a PCR assay for serum HCV RNA should be requested, since up to 15% of patients with HCV may clear the virus spontaneously. The combination of virology and transaminase levels is a useful guide to disease activity and for advice to the patient when attending the clinic.

Consultation

Patients with chronic viral hepatitis are usually asymptomatic. However, some complain of nonspecific complaints such as fatigue, muscle aches, anorexia, right upper quadrant pain and nausea. These symptoms can be debilitating and, in HCV patients, occasionally may warrant antiviral treatment irrespective of disease severity as assessed by liver biopsy. In patients who present later, symptoms and signs of chronic liver disease can occur, although even those chronic viral induced cirrhosis may be asymptomatic.

Patients with HBV or HCV cirrhosis can have extra-hepatic manifestations of disease. In both HBV and HCV, these disorders are thought to be mediated by circulating immune complexes. They occur in 10–20% of patients with chronic HBV infection and in up to 40% of HCV patients (see *Box 13.1*)

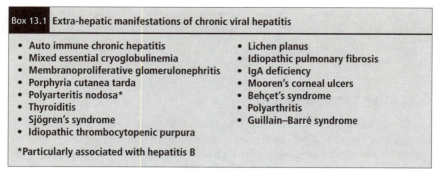

Box 13.1 Extra-hepatic manifestations of chronic viral hepatitis

- Auto immune chronic hepatitis
- Mixed essential cryoglobulinemia
- Membranoproliferative glomerulonephritis
- Porphyria cutanea tarda
- Polyarteritis nodosa*
- Thyroiditis
- Sjögren's syndrome
- Idiopathic thrombocytopenic purpura

- Lichen planus
- Idiopathic pulmonary fibrosis
- IgA deficiency
- Mooren's corneal ulcers
- Behçet's syndrome
- Polyarthritis
- Guillain–Barré syndrome

*Particularly associated with hepatitis B

Risk factors for acquisition of chronic viral hepatitis should be sought (see *Figure 13.1*). The alcohol history is important since, particularly with HCV infection, a high alcohol intake increases the rate of progression of disease. Clinical examination for signs of chronic liver disease or hepatosplenomegaly is performed, although examination is often normal. Signs of vasculitis should be sought and urinalysis for blood or protein indicative of renal disease is mandatory.

Liver function tests

In patients with chronic HBV, serum transaminase will usually be normal or near normal, unless the patient is in the process of immune clearance of the HBV, when transaminase may be markedly elevated. In patients with chronic HBV infection, the serum transaminase is a relatively good guide to the degree of hepatic inflammation. In patients with chronic HCV, the transaminase within individuals tends to fluctuate from normal to abnormal over time, thus a single value is of limited predictive value with regard to necroinflammatory hepatic activity. Indeed, with chronic HCV infection, 50% of HCV infected patients will have normal transaminase values. However, the majority of these viremic patients will have histological evidence of necroinflammatory liver disease. Nonetheless, higher levels of transaminase are often associated with more advanced histology.

Virology and disease patterns

Chronic hepatitis B

The combination of serum transaminase and HBV serology and serum DNA can distinguish four clinical patterns of chronic HBV infection with differing long-term prognosis and response to antiviral therapy (see *Table 13.1*). The disease pattern in an individual will depend on the stage of chronic viral infection within the host. In common, all patients are positive for HBsAg.

Table 13.1. Chronic hepatitis B (HBV) disease patterns

Disease type	HBsAg	HBeAg	HBeAb	ALT	HBV DNA	Antiviral response
Healthy carrier	+	–	+	Normal	–	Not indicated
Immune tolerant carrier	+	+	–	Normal	++	< 10%
Chronic hepatitis/HBeAg positive	+	+	–	Raised (2–8 ×)	+	30%
Chronic hepatitis/HBeAg negative	+	–	+	Raised (2–8 ×)	+	Response with relapse on cessation

HBsAg, hepatitis B surface antigen; HBeAg, hepatitis B e antigen; HBeAb, hepatitis B e antibody; ALT, alanine transaminase.

'Healthy carrier' (hepatitis B e antibody positive)

In patients who are HBsAg positive and hepatitis B e antibody (HBeAb) positive with normal transaminase, no further serological investigation is required. These patients can be regarded as so-called 'healthy carriers' with immune clearance of HBV and do not require liver biopsy. They have a small increased risk of developing hepatocellular cancer and may be offered outpatient follow-up with AFP measurement and ultrasound of the liver, though the value of screening is uncertain.

Immune-tolerant carrier (hepatitis B e antigen positive with normal alanine transaminase)

Patients who are immune-tolerant (HBeAg positive) with normal transaminase should be monitored on a 6-monthly basis with no antiviral treatment. If there is a flare-up in transaminase that persists, then treatment with interferon or lamivudine should be considered with liver biopsy beforehand to stage disease. This disease pattern is commonly seen in young patients who acquired HBV at birth. Patients are clinically well with near-normal liver transaminase and liver histology. In the young, this phase may continue until the age of 15–25 years old. At this stage, the HBV escapes immune surveillance and thus there is a high viral load with HBeAg positivity.

Chronic hepatitis and hepatitis B e antigen positive

This represents the immune clearance phase of chronic HBV disease. This occurs in infant-acquired disease between the ages of 15 and 35 years, but occurs more rapidly in adult-acquired disease. The immune system reacts to the HBV, leading to low levels of viral replication (low levels of HBV DNA and but still HBeAg positive) and immune-mediated liver damage with a chronic hepatitis often with lobular inflammation with raised serum transaminase. Clinically, this is often asymptomatic, although clinical exacerbations of symptomatic 'hepatitis' occur with major elevation of transaminase and raised titers of IgM anti-HBc. Thus, immune clearance may be misdiagnosed as acute HBV. The AFP may also be elevated, leading to concerns regarding hepatoma development. During this phase, 30% of patients will respond to antiviral therapy, but it should be noted that spontaneous HBeAg clearance increases to an annual rate of 10–20%. The transition from replicative to nonreplicative infection may be rapid with little hepatic injury and a reduced chance of cirrhosis developing, or prolonged with recurrent exacerbations of hepatitis, which makes the development of cirrhosis more likely.

Chronic hepatitis with no hepatitis B e antigen

In some European patients, chronic hepatitis with raised transaminase and necroinflammatory changes on liver biopsy is observed, despite the presence of HBeAb or no HBeAg. Many of these patients will have a high viral HBV DNA load. This is often due to infection with a precore HBV mutant that cannot produce HBeAg, which escapes immune surveillance and thus can cause continuing liver damage. A number of other mutants have been described, in particular those with mutations in the pre-S and S regions of the HBV genome. An alternative explanation, in the presence of low or no HBV DNA, is coinfection with HCV or the hepatitis delta virus (HDV). Thus, serum HCV RNA and serology for HDV should be requested. Liver biopsy to stage disease and exclude nonvirological causes of chronic hepatitis should be performed.

Chronic hepatitis C

The disease pattern in chronic HCV can be determined by PCR for serum HCV RNA and staging liver biopsy. Liver histology is of use to decide if antiviral treatment is indicated. The histology activity index is based on the grade of necroinflammation (1–18) and stage of fibrosis (1–6; see *Table 13.2*). Patients may have mild (total score < 6) or moderate/severe chronic hepatitis (score 6 or greater). Patients with a fibrosis score of 6/6 have cirrhosis, irrespective of necroinflammatory score. The presence of moderate fibrosis is predictive of progressive disease.

Table 13.2. Liver histology and chronic hepatitis C (HCV)

Mild chronic HCV infection
Fibrosis score < 2/6
Necroinflammatory score < 3/18
Moderate or severe chronic HCV infection
Fibrosis score > 3–5/6 and/or
Necroinflammatory score is greater than 3/18
Cirrhotic HCV infection
Fibrosis score 6
Variable necroinflammatory score

Spontaneous clearance of HCV

Approximately 15% of patients infected with HCV will spontaneously clear the virus (HCV antibody positive and HCV RNA negative). In patients with a normal transaminase, repeat PCR for serum HCV RNA at 6 months is performed. Provided patients remain well with a normal transaminase and serum HCV RNA negative, then no further investigation is required. The long-term outlook for these patients should be good.

Mild disease

This serum HCV RNA positive cohort represents about 25% of patients presenting with HCV infection. These patients may have slowly progressive disease that will not affect their life expectancy or general health. Unless patients have severe symptoms then it is probably appropriate not to treat this cohort of patients. We review these every 6 months, with repeat liver biopsy every 2–3 years or if there is flare-up in transaminase levels of greater than two to three times the upper limit of normal. If the biopsy reveals worsening necroinflammatory disease and/or fibrosis, treatment should then be considered.

Moderate to severe disease and cirrhosis

These patients with marked fibrosis and positive serum HCV RNA represent those with progressive HCV infection and should be offered antiviral treatment. Patients with compensated cirrhosis should also be offered antiviral treatment, as this may modify disease progression.

Treatment of chronic hepatitis B

The main aim of treatment for chronic HBV is to suppress HBV replication before there is irreversible liver damage. In patients who are HBeAg positive with a raised serum transaminase, there is a loss of HBeAg of 10% per annum and HBeAg seroconversion of 5%. Interferon alpha (IFNα) and the reverse transcription inhibitor lamivudine are effective treatments for chronic HBV infection.

Interferon

IFNα has predominantly antiviral effects. IFNα treatment is most effective in patients with active viral replication and hepatic inflammation (see *Box 13.2*). Previously it

Box 13.2	Indications for interferon treatment of chronic hepatitis B

- Hepatitis B surface antigen positive for more than 6 months (chronic hepatitis)
- Hepatitis B e antigen and hepatitis B DNA positive (active viral replication)*
- Elevated serum alanine transaminase concentration (× 2 upper limit of normal)*
- Moderate/severe chronic hepatitis on liver biopsy

*A low viral load with elevated transaminase are the two factors that are most predictive of response to interferon treatment.

was thought that Asian patients poorly responded to IFNα treatment, but recent studies suggest that they will respond similar to European patients, provided a raised transaminase is present. Treatment should be considered in patients who are HBsAg positive and raised transaminase, or in HBV cirrhosis.

> **Box 13.3 Contraindications to the use of interferon**
>
> - History of suicidal tendency
> - Active psychiatric illness
> - Autoimmune illness, e.g. autoimmune thyroiditis
> - Severe leukopenia or thrombocytopenia
> - Decompensated cirrhosis

Interferon dose regime

IFNα is usually administered as subcutaneous injections in doses of 10 MU three times a week for 16 weeks. Contraindications to treatment are outlined in *Box 13.3*. There is no additional benefit from either steroid pretreatment to induce a rise in ALT or prolongation of the duration of treatment. Patients should be monitored monthly for exacerbation of hepatitis and for side-effects (see *Box 13.4*).

Treatment response

A meta-analysis of placebo-controlled randomized trials of IFNα treatment of chronic HBV showed that 6–12 months after IFNα completion there was:

- 33% loss of HBeAg (12% in placebo)
- 37% loss of HBV DNA (17% placebo)
- 8% loss of HBsAg (2% placebo)

> **Box 13.4 Side-effects of interferon**
>
> - Initial flu-like syndrome, fatigue, anorexia and nausea,
> - Neuropsychiatric depression, paranoia, severe anxiety and psychosis
> - Bone marrow suppression
> - Hair loss
> - Weight loss
> - Induction of an autoimmune hepatitis/thyroid disease
> - Induction of other autoimmune diseases including diabetes, thrombocytopenia, hemolytic anemia, psoriasis, vitiligo, rheumatoid arthritis, systemic lupus erythematosus-like syndromes, primary biliary cirrhosis and sarcoidosis
> - Renal disease: interstitial nephritis, nephrotic syndrome and acute renal failure

In addition, IFNα treatment was found to increase the likelihood of HBeAb seroconversion and normalize transaminase. Interferon should not be used in immune-tolerant carriers and healthy carriers and probably is not indicated in patients with chronic hepatitis and negative HBeAg (see *Box 13.5*) In this latter cohort, patients are probably more suitable for lamivudine treatment.

Interferon treatment of hepatitis B cirrhosis

In patients with compensated cirrhosis, IFNα treatment can be effective and is safe. However, IFNα treatment can

> **Box 13.5 Inappropriate use of interferon treatment for chronic hepatitis B**
>
> - Immune tolerant carrier: normal alanine transaminase (ALT) and hepatitis B e antigen (HBeAg) positive
> - 'Healthy carriers': normal ALT and HBeAg negative
> - Chronic hepatitis with negative HBeAg but raised ALT and hepatitis B DNA (relapse common after interferon)

be associated in 30% of cases with an immune-mediated rise in ALT sometimes associated with loss of HBeAg. This can precipitate decompensation of advanced liver disease.

IFNα treatment of decompensated cirrhosis should ideally be performed in the setting of a tertiary/liver transplantation center. IFNα treatment can improve liver function but is also associated with sepsis and induction of liver failure, which may be severe enough to warrant transplantation.

Treatment of children with chronic HBV

Some children who acquire HBV by vertical transmission will have a raised ALT. This cohort responds in a similar manner to adults whilst those with normal ALT are poor responders. These patients should be referred to a pediatric hepatologist.

Long-term effects of IFN

In general, loss of HBeAg is sustained and, in Europeans, usually followed by a loss of HBsAg and at the same time HBV DNA becomes undetectable by PCR. In Asians, the loss of HBsAg is less frequent, although sustained loss of HBeAg is the general rule.

Lamivudine

Lamivudine inhibits the reverse transcription of HBV DNA. Lamivudine monotherapy for 12 months is effective in suppressing HBV replication and in ameliorating liver disease.

Treatment regime

Currently we would use lamivudine 100 mg o.d. for 1 year in selected patients with chronic HBV (see *Box 13.6*). In patients with renal impairment, dose reduction is required. Patients are followed up monthly with monitoring of full blood count (FBC), electrolytes and liver function. We would measure HBV DNA every 3 months, with HBeAg/Ab status assessed at 9 and 12 months. If patients are still positive, then longer-term treatment can be considered in patients with more advanced liver disease, but only after close discussion with the patient. Further treatment may result in sero-conversion, at the risk of mutant HBV development. After treatment is discontinued, liver function should be measured weekly for the first month in HBeAg-positive patients in case of a hepatitis flare-up, with monthly review for the first 3 months post-treatment cessation for all patients.

> **Box 13.6 Criteria for lamivudine treatment in chronic hepatitis B infection**
>
> - Elevated serum alanine transaminase > 2 × normal
> - Moderate/severe chronic hepatitis on liver biopsy
> - Hepatitis B e antigen (HBeAg) positive (or negative*)
> - Hepatitis B (HBV) DNA positive (viral load > 100 000 copies per ml)
>
> *Lamivudine may be an effective treatment of chronic hepatitis with negative HBeAg as a result of persistent HBV viral replication or precore mutant HBV viral replication

Treatment response

Overall, lamivudine monotherapy for 12 months in patients with active chronic viral hepatitis and HBeAg results positively in approximately 30–35% of patients losing HBeAg, with 15–20% experiencing HBeAg seroconversion. The chance of HBeAg seroconversion increases with duration of treatment and in patients with elevated transaminase before treatment. Sustained seroconversion occurs in 70–85% of cases.

In patients with chronic hepatitis who are HBeAg negative but HBV DNA positive, lamivudine can be used since viral suppression occurs with disease improvement. However, the duration of treatment is unclear because of common relapse, despite patients being negative for HBV DNA by the PCR assay. In patients with aggressive hepatitis, we would use lamivudine long-term to prevent disease progression. If there is clinical deterioration on treatment then referral to a tertiary liver center is recommended for either alternative antiviral treatment or consideration for liver transplantation.

Complications of treatment

Lamivudine-resistant mutants (YMDD motif) arise in up to 30% of cases after 12 months of treatment and 60% of cases after 3 years of treatment. A flare-up in ALT can be associated with the development of mutant HBV. Decompensation can occur in those with advanced liver disease. The development of the YMDD mutant may not interfere with the clinical effectiveness of lamivudine, since 'wild-type' HBV may coexist.

Uncommon adverse effects with lamivudine include pancreatitis and lactic acidosis. An exacerbation of hepatitis can occur on treatment cessation in those that remain HBeAg positive.

Which antiviral therapy to choose

Both IFN and lamivudine are equally efficacious, with HBeAg clearance in a third of patients with chronic hepatitis with a raised ALT. Thus, the decision to use lamivudine or IFNα as primary therapy should be made jointly by the physician and patient. The advantages and disadvantages of each treatment are shown in *Table 13.3*. Lamivudine can be taken orally and has few side-effects, but is associated with resistant HBV mutations of unclear significance. Interferon is taken for a shorter period of time, but is less patient-friendly with regard to route of administration and side-effects. Neither combination treatment of interferon and lamivudine or pretreatment with steroids to induce a rise in transaminase has been shown to be of additional benefit to conventional treatment.

Treatment of chronic hepatitis C

Treatment agents

Monotherapy with either interferon 2α or 2β will result in sustained virological clearance of HBC in about 15–20% of cases. However, combination of interferon

Table 13.3. Advantages and disadvantages of antiviral therapy for chronic hepatits B (HBV)

	Lamivudine		Interferon	
	Advantage	**Disadvantage**	**Advantage**	**Disadvantage**
Duration of treatment		12 months +	4 months	
Route of Administration	Oral			Subcutaneous injection
Side-effects	Minimal			> 20%
HBV mutations		30% at 12 months	None	

with ribavirin is more effective in the treatment of chronic HCV, with improved sustained response rates of approximately 40% and thus represents the treatment of choice. Recently, long-acting interferons, which are attached to a polyethylene glycol molecule (Peg interferon) of either 12 or 40 kD molecular size, have been developed and are more efficacious than standard interferons when administered as monotherapy. The 12-kD Peg interferon 2β, in combination with ribavirin, significantly improves the overall success rate of HCV treatment with marked improvement in the treatment of genotype 1 patients. Similar preliminary results of combination therapy with a 40-kD Peg interferon 2α and ribavirin have recently been published.

Thus, the current treatment of choice for chronic HCV infection is combination therapy for 6–12 months with either standard or Peg interferon and ribavirin.

Indications for treatment

All patients must be HCV RNA positive before treatment is instigated. Any patient with moderate–severe chronic HCV hepatitis on liver biopsy or cirrhosis is suitable for treatment (see *Box 13.7*). Those patients with severe viral symptoms interfering with their lifestyle but mild hepatitis may be offered treatment, although they should be carefully counseled, since they are unlikely to develop severe disease in the long-term. The treatment algorithm for HCV treatment is shown in *Figure 13.2* with specific treatment for the differing HCV disease groups outlined below.

> **Box 13.7 Indications for antiviral treatment in chronic hepatitis C**
>
> - Hepatitis C polymerase chain reaction positive
> - Moderate disease or cirrhosis
> - Mild disease with either systemic symptoms or extraintestinal manifestations

Treatment response

Response to antiviral treatment is based on serum HCV RNA, although serum transaminase can be used as a crude surrogate marker. Sustained response can be defined as those patients who remain serum HCV RNA negative 6–12 months after completing treatment. Relapsers are those patients who initially became serum HCV RNA negative on treatment but subsequently become HCV RNA

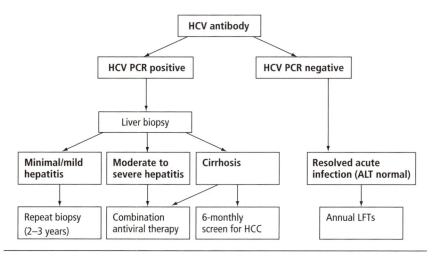

Figure 13.2. Treatment algorithm for HCV treatment

positive when treatment was discontinued. Nonresponders are those who remain PCR positive for serum HCV RNA after 3–6 months of treatment. These patients are very unlikely to respond to further treatment.

Treatment of moderate disease

Combination therapy is the first line treatment for moderate HCV disease. These patients should be subdivided into those who are genotype 1 and non-genotype 1, since controlled trials suggest that genotype 1 patients generally require a longer duration of treatment than non-genotype 1 patients and have a differing response to conventional and Pegylated interferon.

Currently we recommend a regime of 12 months of Peg interferon 2β (12 kD) at a dose of 1.5 μg kg^{-1} week^{-1} and ribavirin (800–1200 mg according to body weight) in patients with HCV genotype 1. This should result in a sustained response rate of approximately 45%. In combination with ribavirin, Pegylated interferons appear to be superior to non-Pegylated interferon in the treatment of this genotype. Although some centers would recommend 6 months of treatment for genotype 1 patients with a low viral load, we believe that the nonstandardization of quantitative HCV RNA makes an accurate decision as to who has a low viral load difficult.

In general, non-genotype 1 patients are treated with 6 months of combination therapy. We would use conventional interferon since this seems to be equally effective as Peg interferon in combination with ribavirin. The sustained virological response rates are between 70% and 80% of patients treated. For patients with non-genotype 1 who have two or more risk factors for poor response (see *Box 13.8*), treatment may be continued for 1 year if there is response (negative serum HCV RNA) after 6 months of treatment.

Treatment of cirrhosis

In patients with compensated cirrhosis, combination therapy of interferon and ribavirin is given for 12 months. Peg interferon (40 kD) is more effective than conventional interferon in the treatment of cirrhotic patients, as monotherapy with

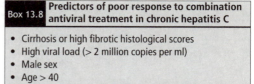

Box 13.8 **Predictors of poor response to combination antiviral treatment in chronic hepatitis C**

- Cirrhosis or high fibrotic histological scores
- High viral load (> 2 million copies per ml)
- Male sex
- Age > 40
- Genotype 1 is the major determinant of poor response to treatment

an overall sustained response rate of over 30% (12% for genotype 1). In the future, treatment with Peg interferon (40 kD) and ribavirin may increase virological response in cirrhotic patients, although confirmatory data for this regime are not available. Although cirrhotic patients have a poorer sustained response rate than noncirrhotic patients, treatment may also reduce the rate of hepatoma development, even if the HCV virus is not cleared. There are little data on the use of antiviral therapy in decompensated HCV cirrhotics.

Treatment of nonresponders and relapsers after interferon monotherapy

Combination therapy is the treatment of choice for relapsers after monotherapy. Six months of combined conventional interferon and ribavirin results in a sustained response rate of almost 50%. In patients who have no virological response to an initial course of interferon, further treatment of IFN alone or in combination with ribavirin is unlikely to lead to response. Nonetheless, if patients are very keen to embark on further treatment, and liver histology has shown progression of disease, then this cohort can be offered a year of combination therapy with Peg interferon and ribavirin irrespective of genotype.

Role of interferon monotherapy

This should be used only in patients who are intolerant of ribavirin or have unstable cardiac disease, anemia, renal insufficiency and those who might conceive on treatment or within 6 months of completing therapy. Peg interferon (either 12 or 40 kD) should be used as this results in an approximate doubling in the sustained virological response compared to conventional interferon monotherapy. Thus, if monotherapy is indicated, we would recommend treatment for 12 months with Peg interferon.

Side-effects *(see Boxes 13.4 and 13.9)*

Although transient or mild side-effects are common during IFN monotherapy, serious toxicity, requiring reduction in dose or cessation of treatment, occurs in 5–10% of patients during treatment. Withdrawal from IFN/ribavirin combination therapy occurs more often, with 10–20% of patients requiring a reduction in dose or cessation of combination therapy. Side-effects, particularly neutropenia (26%) are commoner when Peg interferon 2β and ribavirin are used compared to conventional interferon and ribavirin (14%). The dose reduction schedule for common adverse side-effects is shown in Table 13.4.

Treatment monitoring

The pre-treatment laboratory markers are outlined in *Box 13.10*. Monitoring patients during therapy is extremely important. This requires regular clinical examination, psychological assessment, urinalysis, serum chemistry, blood counts and thyroid function tests. Pregnancy tests should be performed prior to treatment and patients on ribavirin advised not to conceive whilst on treatment and for at least 6 months after combination therapy.

Patients should have a weekly FBC for the first 4 weeks of IFN/ribavirin combination treatment to ensure that the hemolysis that occurs with ribavirin does not cause the hemoglobin to fall below 8 g dl^{-1} in healthy individuals or 10 g dl^{-1} in patients with possible ischemic heart disease. Thereafter, patients are seen on a monthly basis, either by a clinician or a nurse practitioner.

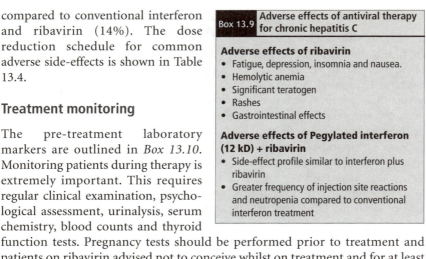

Box 13.9 Adverse effects of antiviral therapy for chronic hepatitis C

Adverse effects of ribavirin
- Fatigue, depression, insomnia and nausea.
- Hemolytic anemia
- Significant teratogen
- Rashes
- Gastrointestinal effects

Adverse effects of Pegylated interferon (12 kD) + ribavirin
- Side-effect profile similar to interferon plus ribavirin
- Greater frequency of injection site reactions and neutropenia compared to conventional interferon treatment

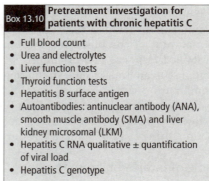

Box 13.10 Pretreatment investigation for patients with chronic hepatitis C

- Full blood count
- Urea and electrolytes
- Liver function tests
- Thyroid function tests
- Hepatitis B surface antigen
- Autoantibodies: antinuclear antibody (ANA), smooth muscle antibody (SMA) and liver kidney microsomal (LKM)
- Hepatitis C RNA qualitative ± quantification of viral load
- Hepatitis C genotype

Outpatient visits

Patients are encouraged to continue treatment and given support for side-effects experienced. Poor compliance with treatment is a major reason for treatment failure, and thus careful supervision of treatment is essential. At each visit, FBC, renal and LFTs should be taken, with 3-monthly thyroid function tests and HCV

Table 13.4. The dose reduction schedule for common adverse side-effects of hepatitis C combination treatment

	50% dose reduction of medication (parentheses)	Stop treatment of interferon and ribavirin
Hemoglobin (g dl^{-1})	< 10.0 (ribavirin)	< 8.5 g dl^{-1}
Total white cell count (× 10^9 l^{-1})	< 1.5 (interferon)	< 1.0
Neutrophil count (× 10^9 l^{-1})	< 0.75 (interferon)	< 0.5
Platelet count (× 10^9 l^{-1})	< 50 (interferon)	< 25

PCR after 3 months of treatment. A negative serum HCV RNA is a positive motivation factor for patients to continue therapy.

Post-treatment

After completing treatment, we recommend follow-up serum transaminase and serum HCV RNA PCR testing at 6 and 12 months. Most patients who remain negative at 12 months will have a sustained response to treatment. We do not perform follow-up liver biopsy after treatment.

Referral for liver transplantation

Any patient with signs of hepatic decompensation, namely elevated bilirubin; ascites, falling albumin (< 35 g dl^{-1}), loss of lean body mass, prolongation of prothrombin time, variceal hemorrhage or hepatic encephalopathy, should be considered for referral to a liver transplantation center. These patients may be suitable for careful antiviral therapy under the supervision of a transplantation center or alternatively need assessment for liver transplantation. Patients with HBV and HCV can be successfully transplanted with results comparable to patients with nonviral causes of liver failure. HBV patients need to have long-term treatment with either HB immune globulin or lamivudine to prevent recurrence of HBV liver disease. In particular, recurrence can lead to rapid deterioration in the liver graft due to fibrosing cholestatic hepatitis. HCV infection recurs in most transplant recipients, although the 5-year survival figures are good. Nonetheless, long-term data on this indolent recurrent disease is uncertain, with late damage to the graft as a result of recurrent infection being a concern.

Further reading

Dienstag, J.L., Schiff, E.R., Wright, T.L., *et al.* (1999) Lamivudine as initial treatment for chronic hepatitis B in the United States. *N. Engl. J. Med.* **341**: 1256–1263.

Fattovich, G., Giustina, G., Degos, F., *et al.* (1997) Morbidity and mortality in compensated cirrhosis type C: a retrospective follow-up study of 384 patients. *Gastroenterology* **112**: 463–472.

Lok, A.S. (1992) Natural history and control of perinatally acquired hepatitis B virus infection. *Dig. Dis.* **10**: 46–52.

Poynard, T., Bedossa, P., Opolon, P. (1997) Natural history of liver fibrosis progression in patients with chronic hepatitis C. The OBSVIRC, METAVIR, CLINICIR, and DOSVIRC groups. *Lancet* **349**: 825–832.

Watson, J.P., Brind, A.M., Chapman, C.E., *et al.* (1996) Hepatitis C virus: epidemiology and genotypes in the northeast of England. *Gut* **38**: 269–276.

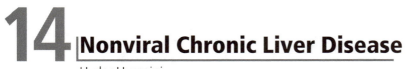

14 Nonviral Chronic Liver Disease

Hyder Hussaini

Introduction

This chapter will deal with the major nonviral chronic liver diseases that present to the outpatient clinic. Specific emphasis is made with regard to diagnosis, management, prognosis and indications for referral for liver transplant assessment.

Nonalcoholic steatohepatitis

Nonalcoholic steatohepatitis (NASH) is a clinical disorder in which patients have the histological changes of alcoholic hepatitis but no history of significant alcohol consumption. An alternative term for this disorder is nonalcoholic fatty liver disease (NAFLD), since patients may not have a hepatic component on liver biopsy, although for the purposes of discussion the term NASH will be used. The pathogenesis of NASH remains unclear, although a sequence of fat accumulation, inflammation and fibrosis is thought to occur.

The histological features of NASH are seen in 7–9% of liver biopsies in the Western world, generally occurring between the ages of 40 and 60, with a female predominance. NASH is associated with obesity (> 70%), rapid weight loss, type 2 diabetes mellitus (35–75%) and hyperlipidemia (20–80%). However, the disorder can occur with none of these factors present. NASH may progress histologically in 40% of cases and be a cause of cryptogenic cirrhosis. The presence of ballooning degeneration, Mallory's hyaline or fibrosis on initial biopsy may predict the late development of cirrhosis in up to 26% of patients over 18 years. However, the risk of cirrhosis seems to be low if the initial biopsy shows steatosis alone.

Clinical features

Most patients with NASH are asymptomatic with a raised transaminase and may have hepatomegaly. We perform an abdominal ultrasound prior to the outpatients' visit, which often reveals a 'bright' liver, indicative of diffuse fatty infiltration, although this is a nonspecific finding. We also perform a virological, autoimmune and metabolic screen for liver disease prior to outpatients with a request for thyroid function test, cholesterol and blood glucose. In the clinic, particular emphasis on alcohol intake is key to making the diagnosis of NASH. A positive diagnosis can be made without liver biopsy. However, we suggest biopsy in most patients (*Box 14.1*), since biopsy is probably the best guide to long-term prognosis.

Management

In patients who are overweight, gradual weight loss is recommended aiming for 5 kg weight loss over 6 months. Rapid weight loss can exacerbate NASH. Metabolic abnormalities of diabetes and hyperlipidemia should be corrected, including the use of statin agents for hypercholesterolemia.

Box 14.1	Indications for liver biopsy in nonalcoholic steatohepatitis patients

- Peripheral stigmata of chronic liver disease
- Splenomegaly
- Thrombocytopenia
- Abnormal iron studies
- Diabetes and/or significant obesity in an individual over the age of 45
- Alanine transaminase > 2 × upper limit of normal for 6 months

Patients with steatosis alone on liver biopsy are advised with regard to their favorable prognosis and are reviewed annually with LFT measurement. If there is a persistent elevation in transaminase (> 3 × upper limit) then re-biopsy is suggested 5 years later. These patients are often managed in the community.

Patients with fibrosis are followed every 6 months with LFT measurements. The prognosis of these patients is less favorable and particular effort is made to normalize any metabolic abnormalities. Patients are offered a further liver biopsy, 3 years after the index biopsy, to assess disease progression. In patients with progressive disease, agents such as ursodeoxycholic acid, vitamin E or metformin may be beneficial. Metformin use is of particular interest, since it reverses insulin resistance and has recently shown benefit in NASH patients in an uncontrolled study. However, further controlled trials are awaited.

Alcohol-related liver disease

Alcohol-related liver disease (ALD) presents with a variety of clinicopathological syndromes, including asymptomatic patients with fatty liver and steatohepatitis, to patients with end-stage liver failure with established severe fibrosis/cirrhosis.

Risk of alcohol-related liver disease

An intake of 80 g (1 l of wine or 4 pints of beer) of ethanol daily for 10–20 years significantly increases the risk of the development of cirrhosis. Interestingly, an intake of 230 g of alcohol for 20 years is associated with cirrhosis in only 50% of cases; thus, both environmental and genetic factors in addition to the amount of alcohol affect the development of liver disease. There is an increased risk of developing cirrhosis secondary to alcohol use with coexistent chronic HCV infection, female gender and increased body weight.

Assessment of alcohol dependence

Establishment of alcohol intake and recognition that patients may or may not be alcohol dependent is crucial to both diagnosis and treatment, since the cornerstone of long-term management is alcohol abstinence. The CAGE questionnaire (see *Box 14.2*) is an easy to use screening test for alcohol dependency, which uses four 'lifestyle' questions. The CAGE questionnaire will be negative for all four questions in 80% of patients with nonALD, with at least two positive replies in patients with alcohol dependency. Additional clues to alcohol dependency include a family history of alcoholism, loss of driving license due to alcohol use and a history of trauma. Patients who are alcohol dependent need counseling from experts in alcohol abuse.

Diagnosis

In patients with ALD, serum transaminase is usually mild to moderately elevated and rarely greater than 400 IU l^{-1}. The AST/ALT ratio, if > 2.0, is suggestive of ALD. Patients may have a raised GGT, although this is not specific to the diagnosis of ALD. A macrocytosis in the blood film, without B_{12} or folate deficiency, can suggest a diagnosis of ALD but it is also seen in established nonalcoholic liver disease. Similarly, thrombocytopenia can arise because of marrow toxicity or hypersplenism. IgA can be elevated in patients with alcoholic hepatitis. Liver biopsy in patients with a history of excess alcohol is of use to stage liver disease, assess for alcoholic hepatitis and give long-term prognostic information.

Clinicopathological syndromes

Alcohol-related fatty liver

Most patients are asymptomatic, some may have mild tender hepatomegaly, transaminase is normal or mildly elevated and jaundice very rare. Although fatty liver can occur with a single alcohol binge, it is more common with prolonged excess alcohol intake and can progress directly to fibrosis, cirrhosis (8–20%) or alcoholic hepatitis (10–35%).

Alcoholic hepatitis

These patients will rarely directly present to outpatients, acute admission being more common. The characteristic presentations of alcoholic hepatitis are of fever, hepatomegaly, jaundice and anorexia. Ascites occurs in 30%, due to portal hypertension, and variceal hemorrhage can occur. Alcoholic hepatitis can occur in the presence of underlying cirrhosis, and may be suggested by the presence of stigmata of chronic liver disease.

Cirrhosis

The clinical features of cirrhosis in ALD are similar to other causes of cirrhosis, although patients may have a coexisting alcoholic hepatitis. Prognosis is determined by the degree of hepatic synthetic dysfunction.

Coexisting liver disease

Although the diagnosis of ALD on history and clinical features may be straight-forward, coexistent disease or alternative diagnoses can occur.

In particular, chronic HCV infection can coexist in 25–65% of patients with a history of alcohol abuse. Co-existent HCV infection is associated with increased disease severity, risk of hepatocellular cancer and reduced survival. Thus, HCV antibody testing and, if needed, HCV RNA measurement is mandatory in all patients with ALD.

Genetic hemochromatosis (GH) is common and can also accelerate the progression of ALD. Unfortunately, serum ferritin is frequently elevated in ALD, since this is an acute phase protein. Similarly, transferrin saturation can be greater than 60%, possibly due to impaired hepatic transferrin synthesis. Thus, genetic studies and liver biopsy to determine the pattern of iron distribution within the liver may be required.

Management

Abstention from alcohol is the key factor in improving disease prognosis. Support from medical staff and alcohol counselors is essential, with entry if needed into alcohol rehabilitation programs if alcohol dependent. Adequate nutrition with B vitamin supplementation and thiamine may be required. No definite benefit from pharmacological intervention has been demonstrated in clinical trials with propylthiouracil, S-adenosylmethionine or colchicine. In patients with histological evidence of alcoholic hepatitis (a Maddrey index > 32 and no signs of bacterial sepsis), we will treat with prednisolone (30 mg day^{-1}) for 1 month, although this remains controversial.

Liver transplantation is effective in alcohol-related cirrhosis with a 1-year survival rate of 90% and is similar to transplantation for nonalcohol-related disease. In general, a 6-month period of alcohol abstention is recommended, mainly to determine the reversible component of ALD, but it may also predict those patients likely to abstain post-liver transplantation. Patients who have been abstinent from alcohol for more than 6 months and still have moderate hepatic impairment (Child B disease) should be referred to a transplantation center for assessment. Patients who are nonalcohol dependent, and who have little comorbid disease, especially myocardial dysfunction, have a better prognosis following transplantation. It is of interest that, although alcohol recidivism is common post-transplantation, it is seldom a cause for graft failure, since most patients will only drink moderately. Some patients who present for the first time with advanced liver disease (Child C) or acute alcoholic hepatitis, particularly if young, should be discussed with transplantation center. However, liver trans-plantation for patients with alcoholic hepatitis is uncommon, because of concerns regarding alcohol use post-transplantation, inability to assess psycho-logical and comorbid disease preoperatively together with the problems of trans-plantation in patients with severe hepatic impairment.

Prognosis

Continued alcoholic intake adversely affects prognosis with more rapid progression of liver disease to cirrhosis and increased mortality. Conversely, abstinence is association with improvement in liver histology, even with advanced disease and reduced complications from varices or ascites.

Approximately 17% of patients with a fatty liver at presentation who continue to drink will develop severe fibrosis/cirrhosis over 10 years, whilst less than 2% who abstain will develop progressive disease. In patients with histological alcoholic hepatitis, 40–50%, will develop cirrhosis over 3 years, although alcohol abstention reduces this proportion to about 18%. In the presence of cirrhosis, an increased inflammatory infiltrate, particularly with neutrophils, is indicative of poor prognosis. A recent UK study showed that the 10-year survival for patients with alcohol-related steatosis was 72%, hepatitis 57%, active cirrhosis 49% and inactive cirrhosis 40%.

The Child classification (see *Table 7.2*) can assist in prognosis in compensated patients. A patient with Child's C disease has a 2-year prognosis of 35%. The Maddrey score (see *Box 14.3*) is useful in the prediction of disease severity and prognosis in acute alcoholic hepatitis. A Maddrey score of greater than 32 is associated with a 35–45% 1-month mortality in patients with alcoholic hepatitis varying with the presence or absence of encephalopathy.

Box 14.3	The Maddrey index

- Discriminate index = (4.6 × [prothrombin time (PT) – control PT]) + (serum bilirubin/17)
- Serum bilirubin is measured in μmol
- Index > 32 = > 35% mortality without encephalopathy at 1 month
- Index > 32 = > 40% mortality with encephalopathy at 1 month

Autoimmune hepatitis

Autoimmune hepatitis is a chronic hepatitis characterized by hyperglobulinemia, circulating autoantibodies and interface hepatitis (piecemeal necrosis) on liver histology. Autoimmune hepatitis can be classified by the circulating autoantibodies associated by the disorder (see *Table 14.1*), although these antibodies are markers rather than the cause of disease.

Table 14.1. Classification of autoimmune hepatitis

	Typical autoantibody pattern	Associated antibodies that may be present
Type 1	ANA >1:320 SMA >1:320	Anti SLA + AMA + p-ANCA +
Type 2	Anti LKM 1 +	Anti SLA +
Sero-negative	Negative ANAs Negative SMAs Negative anti-LKM-1	Anti SLA +

ANA, antinuclear antibody; SLA, antibody to soluble liver antigen; SMA, smooth muscle antibody; p-ANCA, perinuclear antineutrophil cytoplasmic antibody; LKM, liver kidney microsomal antibody.

Classification

Two distinct forms of autoimmune hepatitis exist in addition to seronegative autoimmune hepatitis. Type 1 is the classical autoimmune hepatitis, characterized by antinuclear antibodies (ANAs) and/or smooth muscle antibodies (SMAs). ANA-positive patients may have antibodies directed against single-stranded (anti-ssDNA) and double-stranded (anti-dsDNA) DNA. Titers of greater than 1:320 are usually significant, with titers less than 1:80 being of uncertain significance. Type 2 autoimmune hepatitis is characterized by the presence of antibodies to liver/kidney microsomes (LKM-1) and found in young girls and women with autoimmune hepatitis. Seronegative autoimmune hepatitis is a chronic hepatitis with histological features of autoimmune liver disease and raised immunoglobulins, but is negative for ANAs, SMAs, antimitochondrial (AMA) and LKM antibodies. However, these patients respond to steroid treatment. A proportion of these patients will have circulating antibodies that are not conventionally screened for by immunology laboratories. These include antibodies to soluble liver antigens (SLAs). These antibodies were thought to represent a third class of autoimmune hepatitis (type 3). However, SLA antibodies are found in both type 1 and type 2 autoimmune hepatitis.

Overlap syndromes

Two conditions occur were histological features of either autoimmune hepatitis and/or primary biliary cirrhosis (PBC) occur with noncompatible serology. The 'overlap syndrome' has been described as patients with the histological findings of autoimmune hepatitis, but an isolated rise in AMAs. Autoimmune cholangiopathy (autoimmune cholangitis or immune cholangiopathy) is characterized by histology compatible with PBC in the absence of circulating AMAs, but positive serology for ANAs and/or SMAs.

Clinical features

Patients may present asymptomatically, with elevated transaminase compared to those with acute liver failure, and transaminase greater than 1000 IU l^{-1}, raised prothrombin time and jaundice. Autoimmune hepatitis can be associated with other diseases such as hemolytic anemia, idiopathic thrombocytopenic purpura, type 1 diabetes mellitus, thyroiditis and UC. Diagnosis is made on the combination of immunology and liver biopsy. The differential diagnosis includes acute viral hepatitis, drug-induced hepatitis and chronic HCV (see *Table 14.2*).

Management

All patients with symptomatic autoimmune hepatitis are offered treatment irrespective of histological staging of disease. Those who are asymptomatic with minimal inflammation can be monitored carefully with staging liver biopsies for evidence of disease progression without treatment. In contrast, patients with

Table 14.2. Differential diagnosis for autoimmune hepatitis

Differential diagnosis	Investigation
Chronic hepatitis C (HCV) infection	LKM antibodies and raised immunoglobulins
	HCV RNA+
Acute viral hepatitis	Serology for hepatitis A, B and E
	EBV serology
PBC and PSC	Loss of bile ducts + biliary inflammation
	Periductular fibrosis
	Increased copper associated protein
	AMA/ANCA positive
Drug-induced hepatitis	Clinical history
	Increased eosinophilic infiltrate

LKM, liver kidney microsomal antibody; EBV, Epstein–Barr virus; PBC, primary biliary cirrhosis; PSC, primary sclerosing cholangitis; AMA, antimitochondrial antibody; ANCA, anticytoplasmic antibody.

severe inflammation and significant fibrosis should be treated. The 10-year survival for patients without cirrhosis is approximately 90%, although for those with cirrhosis at presentation survival falls to 50% at 12 years.

Patients are counseled with regard to the duration of treatment and agents to be used. We commence prednisolone (30 mg day^{-1}) for the first month of treatment and then start azathioprine (2 mg kg^{-1}) after 1–2 months as guided by biochemical remission. The prednisolone dose can be tapered usually over 2 months to a maintenance dose of 5–10 mg day^{-1} in combination with azathioprine.

Remission

Normalization of transaminase and serum globulins suggest remission. Histological improvement with inactivity or mild activity confined to the portal tract may lag behind biochemical improvement and antibody titers do not correlate with disease activity.

Maintenance therapy

Our practice is to repeat liver biopsy after 6–18 months of combination therapy in patients, depending on the severity of presentation. If there is minimal inflammation on biopsy, then prednisolone is withdrawn, with maintenance treatment with azathioprine (2 mg kg^{-1}) alone. This is then continued on a lifelong basis, since most patients will relapse within 18 months, particularly if cirrhosis was present on initial liver biopsy. However, there is recent evidence that relapse may be less likely on immunosuppression withdrawal in patients who remain in remission after 4 years of treatment. Thus, we currently counsel patients with regard to the careful withdrawal of immunosuppression after 4 years in remission, provided a staging liver biopsy shows no inflammation or established cirrhosis. In those who do not respond to treatment, second-line immunosuppressant agents are use (see below).

Treatment failure

Up to 20% of patients with autoimmune hepatitis fail to respond to treatment with sustained inflammation on biopsy, or cirrhosis, with progressive liver failure. Treatment failure is more likely in younger patients, LKM-1 positive patients, certain human leukocyte antigen (HLA) phenotypes (HLA-B8 and/or HLA-DR3) and those that present with cirrhosis. Treatment with cyclosporin, methotrexate, mycophenolate–mofetil and 6-MP are possible alternative treatments. Patients should be considered for transplantation if liver function continues to deteriorate.

Primary biliary cirrhosis

PBC occurs mainly in women and rarely below the age of 30, with an incidence in the UK of 32 cases per million. Approximately 50% of patients are asymptomatic at diagnosis, with fatigue, pruritus and arthropathy being common features (see *Box 14.4*) in symptomatic patients.

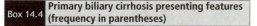

| Box 14.4 | Primary biliary cirrhosis presenting features (frequency in parentheses) |

- Fatigue (50%)
- Pruritus (30%)
- Skin hyperpigmentation (25–50%)
- Musculoskeletal symptoms (40%)
- Sjögren's syndrome (60%)
- Crest syndrome (5–15%)

Natural history

The rate of progression of PBC is variable, although most asymptomatic patients develop symptoms within 4 years of presentation. Asymptomatic patients have a median survival of 16 years, in contrast to symptomatic patients with a median survival of 7.5 years. A progressive rise in bilirubin (> 100 μmol l^{-1}), and a decline in liver synthetic function, are good markers of declining function and should prompt referral for transplant assessment. Hepatoma occurs in 6% of patients with advanced fibrosis or cirrhosis. Portal hypertension can complicate early PBC but in itself is not an indication for transplantation.

Diagnosis

The presence of elevated serum ALP and serum IgM with positive M2 antimitochondrial is diagnostic of PBC. The presence of AMAs alone is a predictor of the eventual development of PBC with greater than 70% of asymptomatic patients with normal LFTs developing symptoms or cholestatic LFTs 10 years later. In asymptomatic patients, we feel that liver biopsy is not indicated since the

| Box 14.5 | Four histological stages of primary biliary cirrhosis |

- Stage zero – normal liver
- Stage one – inflammation and/or abnormal connective tissue confined to the portal areas
- Stage two – inflammation and/or fibrosis confined to portal and periportal areas
- Stage three – bridging fibrosis
- Stage four – cirrhosis

prognosis of early PBC is poorly predicted by liver biopsy. However, in symptomatic patients, the presence of bridging fibrosis/cirrhosis (see *Box 14.5*) is of use in assessing prognosis and to assess hepatoma risk.

Management

Nutritional and metabolic complications of chronic cholestasis

Early in PBC, most patients under follow-up will not be jaundiced and thus vitamin deficiency due to decreased bile acid secretion is relatively rare. However, symptoms of diarrhea can occur in patients due to associated pancreatic insufficiency or celiac disease. These patients should have pancreatic function tests and EMABs requested and treated if appropriate with pancreatic supplements (Creon) and gluten-free diet.

In jaundiced patients, medium-chain triglyceride supplements can be useful to treat steatorrhea. All patients with an elevated bilirubin should receive vitamin A (15 000 units day^{-1}) supplementation, and vitamin D supplementation if serum vitamin D is low.

The management of bone disease is discussed in Chapter 7 (section on Outpatient follow-up for complications of cirrhosis). In the absence of additional risk factors for heart disease, hyperlipidemia should not be treated, since atheromatous disease in PBC is extremely rare.

The symptom of fatigue is common and should prompt investigation with thyroid function tests (20% of PBC patients are hypothyroid) and EMABs. Patients with clinical depression can be safely treated with antidepressant therapy.

Pruritus

Pruritus associated with intrahepatic cholestasis is common, although the etiology is unclear. Accumulation of bile acids or an increase in the concentration or activity of endogenous opioids may be responsible.

Simple emollients such as calamine and antihistamines orally can be effective for mild symptoms. Cholestyramine (4–16 g day^{-1}) binds to bile acids in the gut and is effective, but poorly tolerated with symptoms of bloating and constipation. The use of cholestyramine with sorbitol (Questran light®) can obviate symptoms of bloating. Opioid antagonists such as intravenous naloxone (0.2 μg kg^{-1} min^{-1}) or oral naltrexone (50 mg day^{-1}) are effective in about 25–50% of cases. Rifampicin (300–600 mg day^{-1}) is also effective although drug-induced hepatitis or idiosyncratic reactions can occur. Ursodeoxycholic acid (UDCA) is sometimes effective in controlling pruritus, although many patients with PBC have no response to UDCA treatment. Phototherapy with ultraviolet light (UV-B) alters skin sensitivity to bile acids or alternative agents that lead to pruritus. This treatment has been reported to improve cholestatic pruritus in 1 week. For patients with refractory itch, we have found marked benefit with this modality of treatment. Liver transplantation may be required in patients with cholestatic liver disease whose pruritus is refractory to other interventions.

In our practice for mild pruritus, calamine lotion and piriton are used as first-line agents. Cholestyramine, UDCA and rifampicin are second-line agents. Opioid antagonists and phototherapy are used for resistant cases.

Portal hypertension

IDA can complicate PBC, even early in disease. Some PBC patients can have severe portal hypertension, despite good liver function and no cirrhosis on biopsy. The portal hypertension is probably secondary to nodular regenerative hyperplasia of the liver. These patients can have major variceal hemorrhage or present with intermittent occult bleeding from portal hypertensive gastropathy. Patients with confirmed IDA should be investigated with gastroscopy, duodenal biopsy (to screen for celiac disease) and colonoscopy.

Disease treatment

Prednisolone, azathioprine, penicillamine are ineffective therapies for PBC. Cyclosporin, colchicine, methotrexate and UDCA improve biochemistry and pruritus. Methotrexate improves symptoms and may improve histology. Only UDCA 13–15 mg day^{-1} delays the progression to end-stage liver disease, enhances survival and is well tolerated. However, the case for UDCA treatment is controversial with some recent meta-analyses suggesting no benefit for UDCA treatment in PBC. UDCA and colchicine may be more effective than UDCA alone. Currently, all patients with symptoms and abnormal LFTs are commenced on UDCA. This is given a single dose at night. In patients with severe symptoms, colchicine (0.6 mg b.d.) is added to UDCA treatment. We do not use methotrexate for the treatment of PBC, in view of its potential toxicity and uncertain benefit.

Primary sclerosing cholangitis

PSC is a chronic progressive disorder characterized by inflammation, fibrosis and stricturing of medium-size and large ducts in the intrahepatic and extrahepatic biliary tree. Although the majority of cases have underlying UC (up to 90%), only 5% of patients with UC or CD have PSC.

Clinical features

Most patients are asymptomatic at diagnosis and are often diagnosed on the combination of a patient with colitis and raised ALP. Early symptoms include fatigue and pruritus. Cholangitis occurs in 10–15% at presentation.

Differential diagnosis

In those patients with no colitis, chronic bacterial cholangitis, ischemic cholangiopathy and AIDS cholangiopathy should be considered. Sclerosing pancreatocholangitis, a steroid-responsive disorder, has been described in patients with chronic pancreatitis who have stricturing disease of both pancreatic and bile ducts. Cholangiography can be normal in a variant of PSC known as small-duct PSC. These patients have histological and biochemical features of PSC, which can progress to classical PSC.

Diagnosis

Most patients will have a raised ALP with or without raised bilirubin, which can vary with episodes of cholangitis. Persistent jaundice following an episode of cholangitis usually indicates more advanced disease. Approximately 30% of PSC patients have hypergammaglobulinemia, 40–50% increased serum IgM levels and 65–80% are positive for p-ANCAs. The diagnosis of PSC is made on cholangiography with characteristic multifocal stricturing and dilation (beading) of intrahepatic and/or extrahepatic bile ducts. We feel that liver biopsy is unhelpful in making the diagnosis of PSC and should not be performed prior to cholangiography or if cholangiography is diagnostic. However, liver histology can be helpful in assessing prognosis in those with clinically progressive disease who may need transplant assessment.

Management

This is directed at problems associated with chronic cholestasis (see Primary biliary cirrhosis: Management) and specifically cholangitis. Recurrent cholangitis may present with symptoms of right upper quadrant pain, fever and/or jaundice.

Episodes of cholangitis are treatable with 7 days of antibiotics; we use ciprofloxacin, amoxycillin or septrin. In patients with frequent recurrent attacks of cholangitis, prophylactic antibiotics seem to be useful. We use low-dose antibiotics on a monthly rotating schedule of septrin, ciprofloxacin and amoxycillin. These patients should be further investigated with an abdominal ultrasound to examine for biliary dilation and either MRCP or ERCP. Recurrent cholangitis may indicate disease progression, but choledocholithiasis and cholelithiasis occurs in 30% of PSC patients, whilst 20% will have dominant biliary strictures. Common duct stones are managed by ERCP. Dominant biliary strictures can be endoscopically stented or dilated with good symptom relief. However, we often discuss individual cases with dominant stricture PSC with a liver transplant referral center because of concerns of cholangiocarcinoma and/or if there is poor response to stenting.

The lifetime risk of cholangiocarcinoma in PSC patients is between 10 and 15%. Patients with IBD and cirrhosis seem to have the greatest risk. Rapid clinical deterioration with jaundice, weight loss and abdominal discomfort, or progressive biliary dilatation associated with a dominant biliary stricture, is strongly suspicious of cholangiocarcinoma. These patients should undergo CT and/or MRI with endoscopic cholangiography with cytological brushing of dominant strictures. However, cholangiocarcinoma can be difficult to diagnose despite imaging, biliary cytology or endoluminal biopsy. The survival of PSC patients with cholangiocarcinoma is poor with only 10% surviving 2 years. Unfortunately, liver transplantation is ineffective with all patients eventually developing recurrent disease.

The risk of colon cancer in PSC patients with UC is particularly high. We currently perform endoscopic surveillance in all such patients on an annual basis.

Prognosis

Although the median survival after diagnosis for PSC is 12 years, the course of the disease within individuals is very variable. Patients with Child's C disease have a 7-year survival rate of 25%. The Mayo risk score (see *Box 14.6*) appears to accurately predict survival. A Mayo score of 5 or greater indicates that less than 50% will survive 1 year. In our practice patients with Child C disease and those who have failed medical treatment for recurrent cholangitis, symptomatic cholestasis (including pruritus and lethargy) or who have rapidly progressive jaundice are referred for transplant assessment.

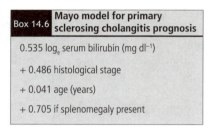

Box 14.6 **Mayo model for primary sclerosing cholangitis prognosis**

0.535 log$_e$ serum bilirubin (mg dl^{-1})

+ 0.486 histological stage

+ 0.041 age (years)

+ 0.705 if splenomegaly present

Hemochromatosis

GH is a disorder in which there is increased iron accumulation resulting in iron deposition particularly in the liver, pancreas and heart. Mutations in the HFE gene on chromosome 6 alter the intestinal transferrin receptor and lead to increase intestinal iron absorption. The prevalence rate for Caucasians for the HFE gene mutation is 1:10 for heterozygotes and 3–5 per 1000 for homozygotes. GH is rare in patients of African descent, but has been reported, although the genetic markers for disease have not been identified.

Clinical features

The majority of patients diagnosed with GH are asymptomatic, because of diagnosis on routine biochemistry with HFE gene analysis. However, symptoms of lethargy and fatigue are common, with arthralgia. Presentation with cirrhosis, pigmentation and diabetes is rare. Hepatocellular carcinoma occurs in cirrhotic GH patients (25% over 20 years) but not in noncirrhotic patients. Diabetes (50% of GH patients) and dilated cardiomyopathy with conduction defects also occur in GH and may respond to venesection, although GH arthropathy poorly responds to iron removal. Hypogonadism leading to libido loss is usually secondary to hypopituitism and can be reversed by venesection. Hypothyroidism, extrahepatic cancers and increased susceptibility to infections such as *Listeria* and *Yersinia* have been reported.

Investigations

Diagnosis of iron overload

The diagnosis of iron overload is generally made by serum measurement of a fasting transferrin saturation (> 50%) and ferritin (> 200 μg l⁻¹) in 90% of patients with GH. The upper limit for these tests is greater in men than in women because of the protective effect of menstrual loss in women. An elevated transferrin saturation is a more specific (90% for C282Y homozygotes) test for iron overload than elevated ferritin (80% for C282Y homozygotes) and thus more useful in screening for GH. Serum ferritin is elevated in chronic viral hepatitis, alcoholic liver disease and nonalcoholic steatohepatitis, in addition to inflammatory diseases such as rheumatoid arthritis and malignancy.

The definitive test for the diagnosis of iron overload is liver biopsy demonstrated by Perl's Prussian blue staining of a liver for parenchymal iron. The distribution of iron may be suggestive of primary or secondary iron overload. Although iron content can be quantified in micromoles of iron per gram dry weight of liver, this is not routinely available.

Genetic testing

All patients with biochemical or histological evidence of iron overload should have C282Y and H63D mutation analysis. The homozygotes for the C282Y genotype account for 93–95% of all cases of GH. Up to 60% of compound heterozygotes (C282Y/H63D genotype) may have iron overload. The risk of iron overload and liver disease is small for C282Y heterozygotes (< 10%) and H63D homozygotes (1%). Up to 10% of patients with iron overload may have a 'normal' genotype since there are a number of HFE gene mutations, which are not routinely tested.

Which patients need liver biopsy?

The rationale for liver biopsy in GH is to stage liver disease, rather than make a diagnosis. Those patients with cirrhosis are at greater risk of hepatoma and have more advanced liver disease. Two studies have now shown that homozygotes with the C282Y mutation with normal LFTs, ferritin less than 1000 μg l⁻¹ and no hepatomegaly are very unlikely (100% negative predictive value) to have any hepatic fibrosis. We currently do not biopsy patients with confirmed GH on biochemical and genetic testing, who have normal LFTs, no stigmata of chronic liver disease and a ferritin less than 1000 μg l⁻¹.

Treatment

Therapeutic phlebotomy removes 200–250 mg of iron with each 500 ml of blood venesected, and thus reduces the degree of iron overload. We venesect any patient with biochemical features of iron overload and homozygote (C282Y) for GH, irrespective of age, unless they have comorbid disease that would reduce their life expectancy.

We use the hematology nurses to perform venesection on an outpatient basis, although a GI nurse or phlebotomist are alternative personnel to perform phlebotomy, according to a set protocol. Currently most patients initially undergo removal of one unit of blood per week. In the elderly or those with cardiorespiratory disease, venesection is initially performed every 2 weeks. On this venesection schedule, most patients will achieve normal iron indices within 3–6 months, obviously dependent on their initial degree of iron overload.

Patients undergo regular phlebotomy until iron stores are normalized (serum ferritin concentration < 50 $\mu g\, l^{-1}$ and transferrin saturation < 50%). In general, as ferritin and transferrin saturation starts to fall, the frequency of venesection can be reduced, since many patients find that weekly venesection is inconvenient, particularly if asymptomatic. If the hemoglobin falls below 10 g dl^{-1} then venesection is discontinued for 2–4 weeks. Maintenance venesection with 1 unit removed every 2–4 months is usually sufficient to maintain a normal transferrin saturation and ferritin below 50 $\mu g\, l^{-1}$. Although patients are concerned regarding dietary intake of iron, the key point is to avoid iron supplements and moderate rather than avoid iron-rich food, since the maximal uptake of iron at 1 mg day^{-1} is easily offset by venesection of 1 unit of blood containing 250 mg of iron.

In patients who poorly tolerate venesection, chelation therapy with desferoxamine can lead to clinical improvement. However, smaller amounts of blood (250 ml) venesected less frequently (every 2–3 weeks) usually avoid problems that may be encountered with the conventional venesection schedule.

Screening (see also Chapter 10, Screening for hemochromatosis)

Currently we will only screen for GH in first-degree relatives. If the index case is a homozygote for C282Y, then a fasting sample for serum iron, total iron binding capacity, transferrin saturation and serum ferritin is taken with an EDTA sample for HFE gene analysis from all first-degree relatives. HFE gene analysis is performed if relatives have a raised ferritin or transferrin saturation. In children, to avoid undue distress, we normally advise the spouse to be assessed for HFE gene status and only advise screening of children if the spouse is heterozygous for C282Y. The optimum time for relatives to be screened is between 18 and 30, when biochemical evidence of iron overload is present without organ damage.

Management of heterozygote patients

Although up to 10% of heterozygotes for GH can have biochemical evidence of iron overload, actual liver disease is rare. However, although clinical manifestations of iron overload appear to be quite uncommon, patients who are either postmenopausal women or middle-aged men heterozygous for GH do have an increased risk for cardiovascular disease. The reasons for this are unclear.

Wilson's disease

Wilson's disease is an autosomal recessive disorder with reduced biliary copper excretion resulting in accumulation of copper in the liver and brain. Patients with liver disease can present with abnormal LFTs alone to chronic hepatitis or acute liver failure. Wilson's should be suspected in patients under the age of 30, with the aforementioned clinical presentation.

Diagnosis

Slit lamp examination may detect Kayser–Fleischer rings, which are present in about 50% of all Wilson's disease patients. Although serum ceruloplasmin concentration can be low in Wilson's, a normal ceruloplasmin does not exclude Wilson's disease, since ceruloplasmin is an acute phase protein. Moreover, a low ceruloplasmin is found in 10% heterozygotes with Wilson's disease, acute and chronic liver disease or malabsorptive conditions.

Urinary copper excretion is usually greater than 100 μg in patients with Wilson's disease (normal 20–50 μg day^{-1}). Oral administration of 500 mg of D-penicillamine increases urinary copper excretion to > 1200 μg copper in 24 h compared to normals with less than 500 μg in 24 h. In cases difficult to diagnose, quantitative hepatic copper can be measured and is usually greater than 250 μg of copper per gram of dry weight (normal < 50 μg per gram of dry weight).

Management

Patients with Wilson's disease should be assessed by a dietician with regard to a low copper diet. Penicillamine, at a dose of 1000–2000 mg day^{-1} in four divided doses, is the treatment of choice. Urinary copper excretion should be greater than 2000 μg day^{-1} on treatment, falling to less than 500 μg day^{-1} by 6 months. The dose of penicillamine can then be reduced to maintenance therapy or alternatively oral zinc acetate (50 mg t.d.s.) can be used. On a monthly basis, FBC and urinalysis should be requested. The common side-effects of penicillamine therapy are listed in *Box 14.7*. In patients unable to tolerate penicillamine, trientine, another copper chelation agent, can be used. Prognosis is generally good in treated patients. Screening of first-degree relatives by slit-lamp examination, LFTs, measurement of serum copper and ceruloplasmin, and 24-h urine copper excretion is mandatory.

Box 14.7 Side-effects of penicillamine
• Drug fever and rash – stop treatment for 1 month and restart at 25 mg day^{-1}. Double dose at weekly intervals
• Nausea, vomiting and anorexia – dose reduction
• Aplastic anemia is rare
• Nephrotic syndrome

Further reading

Alvarez, F., Berg, P.A., Bianchi, F.B., *et al.* (1999) International Autoimmune Hepatitis Group report: review of criteria for diagnosis of autoimmune hepatitis. *J. Hepatol.* **31**: 929–938.

Bacon, B.R. and Sadiq, S.A. (1997) Hereditary hemochromatosis: presentation and diagnosis in the 1990s. *Am. J. Gastroenterol.* **92**: 784–789.

Bacon, B.R., Faravash, M.J., Janney, C.G. and Neuschwander-Tetri, B.A. (1994) Nonalcoholic steatohepatitis: an expanded clinical entity. *Gastroenterology* **107**: 1103–1109.

Devlin J. and O'Grady, J.O. (2000) Indications for referral and assessment in adult liver transplantation: a clinical guideline. *BSG Guidelines in Gastroenterology*. British Society of Gastroenterology.

Kaplan, M.M. (1996) Primary biliary cirrhosis. *N. Engl. J. Med.* **335**: 1570–1580.

Lee, Y.M. and Kaplan, M.M. (1995) Primary sclerosing cholangitis. *N. Engl. J. Med.* **332**: 924–933.

Metcalf, J.V., Mitchison, H.C., Palmer, J.M., *et al.* (1996) Natural history of early primary biliary cirrhosis. *Lancet* **348**: 1399–1402.

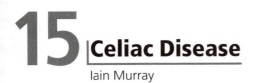

Celiac Disease

Iain Murray

Introduction

Celiac disease is a condition characterized by morphological changes in the proximal small intestine, which improve on the withdrawal of gluten from the diet. This involves avoidance of foods containing wheat, barley and rye. Untreated celiac disease produces a plethora of symptoms including diarrhea, weight loss, iron, folate and B_{12} deficiency.

Epidemiology

There is great geographical variation in prevalence of celiac disease (see *Table 15.1*). The reported prevalence in the UK is 1:1000–1500, although in Belfast a prevalence of 1:152 has been seen based on serological testing. Therefore, a hospital serving a population of 250 000 could expect to treat and monitor at least 170–250 patients with celiac disease, but there will be a further seven undiagnosed celiac patients for every one diagnosed and under follow-up.

Table 15.1. The worldwide prevalence of celiac disease

Country	Prevalence
Denmark	1:10 000
Finland	1:130 or 1:370
Germany	1:463
Holland	1:300
Hungary	1:85
Italy	1:184, 1:400, 1:556 or 1:613
Jordanian Arab	1:2800
New Zealand	1:82
Northern Ireland	1:122 or 1:152
Norway	1:287 or 1:330
Spain	1:389
Sweden	1:189
USA	1:250 or 1:4587
Wales	1:324

Although it was originally believed that celiac disease presented in childhood, it is now appreciated that presentation may be at any age and that presenting features are diverse and often mild. Peak incidences occur at 9 months – 3 years, in the third decade and a smaller peak in the fifth to sixth decades.

Classically a disease of Caucasians, it is also seen in other races. For example, Punjabis and Gujeratis taking a Western diet have a high incidence of celiac disease, which is not revealed when eating their traditional maize-based diet.

The male to female ratio is 1:3 with presentation at earlier age in females. The median delay in diagnosis from commencement of symptoms is 3 years but is frequently much longer.

Cigarette smoking may be protective against the development of celiac disease (odds ratio 0.39). Among active smokers with celiac disease, the age of onset correlates with number of cigarettes smoked, consistent with smoking delaying the development of the disease.

The genetic basis of celiac disease

Celiac disease is often familial, although the genetic basis is not fully determined. Major histocompatibility complex class II alleles DQA1*0501–DQB1*0201 (DQ2) and DQA1*03–DQB1*0302 (DQ8) are strongly associated with the condition (e.g. DQ2 molecule confers a risk of celiac disease among diabetic children of 4.1). HLA-DQ2 is found in 91–93% of celiac patients and 12–18% of controls in Northern Europe. Therefore, although the HLA-DQ2 and DQ8 gene loci are strong risk factors for celiac disease, not all individuals with this genotype will develop the disease. Several non-HLA gene loci probably also play a major role in determining susceptibility to developing celiac disease. A candidate gene on chromosome 6p, 30- cM from the HLA gene has been identified.

Making a diagnosis

Small bowel biopsies

Diagnosis is based on finding the characteristic histological changes on small bowel biopsy, with unequivocal improvement on a gluten-free diet. Most adult gastroenterologists now perform endoscopic biopsy of the second part of the duodenum in preference to jejunal biopsies using dedicated capsules, for example the Crosby capsule. Duodenal biopsies have been shown to be equally effective in diagnosing celiac disease and are easier to perform.

Initial histological changes comprise of an increase in intraepithelial lymphocytes, then an increase in lamina propria inflammatory cells is seen together with crypt hypertrophy and villous atrophy. Villous atrophy is not specific to celiac disease and may be seen in other conditions including tropical sprue, HIV, renal failure, cow's milk intolerance and giardiasis. Hence, both the AGA and the BSG recommend repeat biopsies after a gluten-free diet (for a minimum of 4–6 months).

Many clinicians do not repeat the biopsy if the patient has shown symp-tomatic response to the gluten-free diet, although this can only be recommended where endomysial antibody (EMA) (or tissue transglutaminase, tTG) is positive and initial biopsy is typical of celiac disease. Even in unequivocal celiac disease and with good compliance with a gluten-free diet, the histological changes may not completely reverse within 6 months and can take 24 months to resolve completely. There is no indication for a gluten challenge and third biopsy in adults if histological improvement is unequivocal and symptoms resolve on a gluten-free diet.

When the diagnosis is unclear, a further biopsy while taking a diet containing a minimum of 10 g of gluten per day (four slices of bread) for at least 2 weeks is recommended. In children, this gluten challenge should be for 6 weeks. Failing this, further evidence of the diagnosis should be sought with EMA and antigliadin antibodies. This difficulty in diagnosis most commonly occurs when a patient has commenced a gluten-free diet prior to the initial consultation and the small bowel histology is normal or equivocal.

Symptomatic response to gluten is insufficient to make the diagnosis, as patients with IBS frequently develop increased symptoms after eating wheat. Abdominal symptoms after the consumption of cereals is not uncommon: in one study, 9% had celiac disease, 8% latent celiac disease and 20% allergy to cereals (based on skin prick, patch testing or radioallergosorbent assay).

Self-diagnosis of celiac disease is common, both in patients with IBS and in those who have relatives with celiac disease. HLA genotype suggests that one-third of self-diagnosed individuals with celiac relatives do not have the disease themselves. Since both antibody status and small bowel histology will return to normal in celiac patients with long-term gluten-free diet, dietary trials are best avoided.

The role of small bowel radiology

Small bowel radiology findings equate well with symptom control. Although not usual for routine diagnosis, patients are sometimes referred following an abnormal small bowel contrast study. The typical finding is of reduced jejunal and increased ileal folds (reversed fold pattern) and has a sensitivity of 86–90%.

The role of antibody testing

Antibody testing is used to determine those requiring further investigations by endoscopic duodenal biopsy. IgA EMA are the most sensitive and specific. Their sensitivity is 80–100% and specificity 98–100%. A few studies have found lower sensitivity and specificity, so it is important to know local results for sensitivity and specificity to advise on the need for further investigation. EMAB testing uses indirect immunofluorescence with either monkey esophagus or human umbilical cord as the substrate. There is little difference between the sensitivity and specificity obtained using these substrates.

IgA and IgG antigliadin antibodies may also be used in selecting patients for biopsy. These are detected by ELISA and are less expensive than EMAB testing but their reported sensitivity and specificity varies greatly between laboratories. The sensitivity and specificity of IgA antigliadin is 50–96% and 62–99%, respectively, and for IgG antigliadin is 73–100% and 47–94%, respectively.

With the recognition of tTG as the tissue antigen for EMA commercial kits are available for testing IgA tTG. Quoted sensitivity and specificity is 81–100% and 78–97% with good concordance between this and IgA EMAB testing. Again an ELISA test, it is likely to be cheaper than EMA testing with very slightly reduced sensitivity and specificity.

Immunoglobulins should also be measured in the diagnosis of celiac disease. Selective IgA deficiency is found in 0.4% of the general population and 1.7–4% of celiac patients; 7.7–40% of patients with selective IgA deficiency have celiac disease and are usually IgA EMA, tTG and antigliadin antibody negative (but IgG antigliadin positive).

Because the sensitivity of antibody testing is not 100%, small bowel biopsies should be obtained in any case where the clinical index of suspicion is high, even if antibody testing is negative.

Presenting features

One of the major problems in diagnosing celiac disease is the great diversity of presenting symptoms (see *Box 15.1*). The classic presentation of steatorrhea, weight loss and failure to thrive may be seen in children, but the commonest presentation in adulthood is IDA or general malaise.

Many celiac patients are now diagnosed as a result of screening high-risk groups such as those with insulin-dependent diabetes mellitus or autoimmune thyroid disease. A large number of conditions, mainly autoimmune, are known to be associated with celiac disease (see *Table 15.2*). Screening-detected celiac patients often have suffered from minor symptoms of tiredness, arthralgia or minor abdominal symptoms for years before diagnosis.

GI symptoms are present in 76% at diagnosis; 56% have diarrhea/steatorrhea, 32.7% abdominal pain and 15% constipation. Dyspepsia is more common in celiac disease (the relative risk is twice that of the general population) yet conversely the prevalence of peptic ulcer disease is lower, with reduced HP infection. The reasons for these findings are unknown. Endoscopic appearances of reduced or scalloping of the folds in the second part of the duodenum may lead to biopsy and diagnosis of celiac disease.

Box 15.1	Presenting features of celiac disease

Childhood
- Failure to thrive
- Weight loss
- Abdominal distention
- Muscle wasting
- Diarrhea/steatorrhea
- Hypotonia
- Vomiting
- Constipation
- Rickets

Adults
- Diarrhea
- Iron deficiency
- Weight loss
- Abdominal pain
- Dermatitis herpetiformis
- Folate/B$_{12}$ deficiency
- Mouth ulcers
- Constipation
- Osteoporosis/osteomalacia
- Personality problems
- Screening of high-risk groups (see *Table 15.2*)

Table 15.2. Conditions associated with celiac disease

Condition	Incidence in celiac disease	Celiac disease incidence in patients with these conditions	Comments
Dermatitis herpetiformis	2–5%	72%	A gluten-sensitive enteropathy can be found in most patients with dermatitis herpetiformis. A gluten-free diet (GFD) treats the skin lesions and the dose of dapsone or sulfapyridine can be reduced or discontinued in many
Thyroid disease	20–30%	3.3–4.3%	Most celiac patients with autoimmune thyroid disease are euthyroid or have subclinical hypothyroidism. GFD reverses this or reduces thyroxine requirements
Diabetes mellitus	No increase	2.6–6.45%	No increase in pancreatic β cell auto-immunity in celiac disease. Increase in celiac disease seen in Type I diabetes only
Neurological disease		12.5–17%	Increased incidence in unexplained neurological disorders including 'idiopathic ataxia' with anti-Purkinje antibodies
Down's syndrome		4–18.6%	Most studies report incidence of celiac disease of 6–7%
Pancreatic disease	29–33%	7.1%	High incidence of pancreatic insufficiency in celiac disease at diagnosis improving after 2 months GFD to 6.7%. High incidence of celiac disease in idiopathic pancreatitis
Primary biliary cirrhosis	3%	2.6–7%	Liver function tests do not improve with gluten-free diet
Autoimmune hepatitis		2.8–4%	False-positive IgA antigliadin antibodies are common in many type of chronic liver disease including alcoholic, hepatitis C, primary sclerosing cholangitis and autoimmune liver disease.
Abnormal liver function tests	40–44%	8.6–9.3%	Elevated transaminases reverse on GFD
Turner's syndrome		2.2–10.8%	
Idiopathic dilated cardiomyopathy		5.8%	
Sjögren's syndrome		14.7%	
Microscopic colitis		27%	Lymphocytic colitis definitely associated with celiac: possibly collagenous colitis
Arthritis	26%	0.4–2%	Increased incidence of celiac disease in juvenile chronic arthritis, sacroileitis in bone scan in 64% of celiac patients
Specific enamel defects		7.7%	Aphthous mouth ulcers common in celiac disease
Alopecia areata		1.2%	

The commonest hematinic deficiency is iron deficiency, although both folate and B_{12} deficiencies are common. Six per cent of patients with folate deficiency have celiac disease. Celiac disease is found in 12–14% of symptomatic iron-deficient adults. Although many recover by 6 months with gluten-free diet alone, some remain iron deficient for up to 2 years. Hence, iron supplements should be prescribed until stores are replenished.

Although celiac disease affects the proximal small bowel and B_{12} absorption is from the terminal ileum, B_{12} deficiency is found in 41% of newly diagnosed celiac patients and responds to gluten-free diet alone after 2–13 months. Paresthesia secondary to B_{12} deficiency should be treated by parenteral replacement but this could be discontinued once a gluten-free diet is established.

Treatment

The Dutch physician Dicke first established the relationship between symptoms and the ingestion of wheat. He observed during the war years that children with celiac disease thrived when there was a bread shortage. Their illness recurred when bread became available again. Treatment has altered little since then, although the molecular basis of the reaction to gluten in the diet is better appreciated.

Many foodstuffs contain gluten and it is imperative that a dietitian assesses all patients newly diagnosed with celiac disease. National societies such as The Coeliac Society in Great Britain, compile food directories which list foods known to contain no or minimal quantities of gluten. A 'gluten-free diet' is usually wheat starch-based and contains trace quantities of gluten. Most patients with celiac disease are able to tolerate this without symptoms or small bowel morphological changes.

Prolamins in wheat, barley and rye are responsible for the changes seen in the small bowel. Gluten-free bread tends to be dry and attempts to improve palatability have led to the addition of wheat grain. Likewise, oats do not produce changes in many celiac patients but are often treated at the same mill as wheat, resulting in cross-contamination. Adults with celiac disease can be advised that consuming one portion of oats (50 g) daily from reliable wheat-free sources is unlikely to cause any ill effects. However, they should be told to discontinue oats if symptoms recur. Likewise, oat ingestion in dermatitis herpetiformis does not result in either positive celiac antibodies or small bowel histological changes, although some patients do develop mild rashes.

Dietary studies have found that those compliant with their diet often have reduced lean body mass, low calorie and complex carbohydrate intake with high protein and fat intake, especially saturated fats. A gluten-free diet results in a significant increase in body weight, fat mass, bone mass and BMI but neither lean-tissue nor muscle mass. Calcium, fiber and iron intake is also reduced by those taking a strict gluten-free diet. A dietary assessment should include advice about increasing complex carbohydrates with subsequent reduction in other foodstuffs.

Problems of refractory celiac disease and of assessing and dealing with poor compliance are discussed later.

Associated diseases

Autoimmune disease

Many diseases are associated with celiac disease more commonly than would be expected by chance alone (see *Table 15.2*). These are used to target screening of specific populations for celiac disease and also determine the basis for several of the tests performed during follow-up. The prevalence of other autoimmune diseases with celiac disease is much higher in those diagnosed in later life. Nonspecific low titers of autoantibodies are seen frequently when celiac disease is first diagnosed and disappear with gluten-free diet. It is possible that early diagnosis and treatment of celiac disease may help to prevent the onset of autoimmune disease.

Malignant disease

The incidence of adenocarcinoma of the upper GI tract and of lymphoma of the small intestine is greatly increased in untreated celiac disease (relative risks 7–240 for small bowel adenocarcinoma and 60–876 for small bowel lymphoma). In one study, 4% presented coincidentally with an associated lymphoma. However, 5 years after diagnosis and treatment with gluten-free diet, the incidence is indistinguishable from the general population. The effect of occasional dietary lapses is unclear. Most cases of small bowel adenocarcinoma and lymphoma are diagnosed coincidentally with a new diagnosis of celiac disease. Overall survival of lymphoma with celiac disease is very poor: 31% 1-year and 11% 5-year survival. Survival is particularly poor in those with known celiac disease developing lymphoma rather than diagnosed coincidentally.

Osteoporosis and osteomalacia

Osteoporosis is common in untreated celiac disease. Cases diagnosed through screening have reduced bone densities indistinguishable from those who present with symptoms. The cause may partly be a secondary hyperparathyroidism resulting from reduced calcium and vitamin D absorption. Both peripheral and axial fractures are greatly increased in celiac disease, mostly before diagnosis.

BMD should be measured at diagnosis by DEXA scanning. This is especially important following a fragility fracture, in women at menopause and in men over 55 years of age.

All patients with celiac should be reminded of the importance of a strict gluten-free diet in reducing osteoporosis (an 8% increase in bone density, especially during the first year of treatment). General lifestyle advice should be given including the value of exercise, stopping smoking, avoiding excess alcohol and taking sufficient dietary calcium. Lactase deficiency is common in celiac disease and, unlike other disaccharidase deficiencies, does not respond rapidly to gluten-free diet. This results in a reduced lactose intake including milk and dairy products, and therefore a low calcium intake. A daily intake of 1500 mg calcium is needed. Age and sex determine other treatment (see *Box 15.2*).

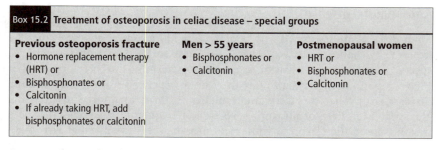

Box 15.2	Treatment of osteoporosis in celiac disease – special groups	
Previous osteoporosis fracture	**Men > 55 years**	**Postmenopausal women**
• Hormone replacement therapy (HRT) or	• Bisphosphonates or	• HRT or
• Bisphosphonates or	• Calcitonin	• Bisphosphonates or
• Calcitonin		• Calcitonin
• If already taking HRT, add bisphosphonates or calcitonin		

A repeat bone density scan is recommended annually after commencing a gluten-free diet in those with initially reduced bone density and in those taking bisphosphonates or calcitonin. Bone density is unlikely to improve after 1 year with diet alone, although bone mineral loss will continue to be less than in those not on the diet. If HRT is used, BMD should be repeated after 10 years and therapy continued if there is still evidence of osteoporosis. If BMD falls more than 4% in 2 successive years, change to a different drug treatment. If BMD is stable, treatment should be for a minimum of 3 years. If drug therapy is stopped, it should be restarted if BMD falls more than 4% per year.

Of celiac patients taking a gluten-free diet, only females diagnosed in adulthood have a reduced BMD compared to age- and sex-matched controls, demonstrating the success of early commencement of a gluten-free diet.

Osteomalacia with celiac disease is much less frequent but is important to diagnose to ensure adequate calcium and vitamin D replacement.

Others

Untreated celiac disease results in delayed menarche, an increase in secondary amenorrhea, spontaneous abortion rate (relative risk 8.9), reduced fetal growth with low birth weight and early menopause. The poor outcome of pregnancy is reversed by a gluten-free diet.

Celiac disease also results in reduced psychological well-being, with higher levels of anxiety and depression, independent of compliance with gluten-free diet.

The role of clinic follow-up

Following diagnosis, patients should be seen by a dietitian and commenced on a gluten-free diet. Membership of national societies (e.g. The Coeliac Society in the U.K.) is strongly recommended. They produce booklets of gluten-free foods, lists of manufacturers, recipe advice and give excellent general support to all celiac patients, particularly those recently diagnosed who often struggle to cope with the dietary restrictions imposed. The Coeliac Society currently has 54 000 members.

Celiac patients should be seen by a gastroenterologist soon after diagnosis to discuss their condition and its excellent prognosis. They need support and advice about the effect of the disease and diet on their health.

Compliance

Compliance is best in those who are well informed. Those who are screening detected may have poorer compliance with diet than those detected as a result of typical symptoms. Teenage years are particularly difficult with many feeling peer pressure to conform being greater than their need for good physical health; 45–81% of teenagers and young adults with celiac disease are fully compliant with their diet but 12–37% take a fully gluten-containing diet. Compliance is better in females, younger children, those with good school grades and those with good self-esteem.

Diagnosis based on two or three biopsies and regular follow-up also improves compliance. Children and adolescents with insulin-dependent diabetes mellitus and celiac disease are less likely to follow a strict gluten-free diet and to have a high saturated fats intake. Following diagnosis in childhood, 64% continue on a completely gluten-free diet into adult life, 24% occasionally take gluten-containing foods and 12% take a fully gluten-containing diet. Those complying with a gluten-free diet often experience social and practical problems. Height and weight may be lower in those not compliant with their gluten-free diet. In some countries, poor compliance may be due to poor food labeling.

Investigations

Individual clinicians will need to decide if they are satisfied with initial histo-logical appearances, symptomatic response to gluten-free diet and autoantibody results. If a repeat duodenal biopsy following commencement of diet is performed, this should be done after 4–12 months, although full histological improvement may take 2 years. Patients should then be followed up at least once per year checking weight, symptomatic response and dietary compliance. Investigations to be performed are listed on *Box 15.3*.

EMABs and antigliadin antibodies become negative after compliance with a gluten-free diet, with 58–77% becoming seronegative after 3 months and 87–100% at 1 year. Although positive antibodies imply gluten ingestion, low quantities of gluten in the diet do not result in positive antibodies (>2 g day^{-1} of gluten will result in positive EMA with lower amounts sometimes resulting in positive antibodies). Antibodies are therefore not a perfect test for compliance and do not predict persisting villous atrophy. Antibodies can become negative before return of the mucosa to normal or persist at low titer, despite return of the small bowel histology to normal.

Because celiac disease is associated with hypoplenism, infection with encapsulated organisms is more likely. Vaccination against pneumococci is recommended in those with evidence of hyposplenism (e.g. raised platelet count), but whether all patients with celiac disease should be vaccinated is not clear. Patients with selective IgA deficiency are more prone to recurrent infection, as well as atopic diseases and silent forms of celiac disease.

Refractory celiac disease

Up to 17% of celiac patients do not respond symptomatically to gluten-free diet. Such patients and those in whom symptoms return despite a gluten-free diet have refractory celiac disease.

Management of refractory celiac disease

A logical stepwise course of investigation should be followed to determine the cause and determine management. The likelihood of complications and local resources will determine the exact order of investigation. In the majority, failure to respond is due to poor dietary compliance and a dietitian should again obtain a full dietary history. Failure of antigliadin and EMABs to become negative, or becoming positive again after being negative, suggests poor compliance.

Assess dietary compliance

'Gluten-free' products include wheat germ, which actually contains trace quantities of gluten: thus WHO/FAO Codex Alimentarius gluten-free products may contain up to 0.3% of protein from gluten-containing grains. Symptoms may resolve in 23% and improve in 45% by switching to a completely gluten-free diet. An elimination diet may improve symptoms in 77% with recurrent symptoms on the addition of foods including amine, salicylate and soy.

However, in studies, the intake of trace amounts of gluten in a gluten-free diet or no gluten was not shown to correlate with persistence of villous atrophy. Wheat starch-based gluten-free flour products do not affect villous architecture, enterocyte height, density of intraepithelial lymphocytes or mucosal HLA-DR expression, nor do they result in detectable serum celiac antibodies. The converse situation also exists, where despite symptomatic response, there is persistent villous atrophy: the significance of this is unknown.

Re-evaluate initial diagnosis and consider ulcerative jejunitis/malignant complications

The original histology should be reviewed and repeat endoscopic duodenal biopsies obtained to determine if there has been any histological improvement. Enteroscopy allows jejunal as well as duodenal biopsies and can diagnose the complications of celiac disease, ulcerative jejunitis and lymphoma. Small bowel radiology and abdominal CT scan may also determine the latter. Enteroscopy has little role to play in uncomplicated celiac disease but is of value both in refractory disease and where the initial duodenal histology is equivocal. Although the disease usually produces more marked changes proximally, in 10% of patients changes in the jejunum are more marked and in a few, may be diagnostic when duodenal biopsies are not.

Consider other coexistent diseases

Lactase deficiency is common in untreated celiac disease and persists for many months after adequate gluten-free diet. In patients taking more than half a pint of milk per day, consideration of a trial of lactose and gluten-free diet should be made or a lactose hydrogen breath test performed.

Other contributing factors can include microscopic colitis, exocrine pancreatic insufficiency, fructose malabsorption, anal sphincter dysfunction and coexistent IBS.

True refractory celiac disease

If the diagnosis is confirmed, compliance is not in doubt and no other cause for failure to respond is identified, then oral steroid therapy may be effective (commencing initially at a dose of 30 mg day^{-1} and titrating the dose to response). This will exacerbate reduced BMD. Methotrexate and azathioprine have also been used in nonresponsive celiac disease to good effect. There is also a case report of the effective use of elemental diet.

Complications of refractory celiac disease

Ulcerative jejunitis has been viewed as a premalignant condition, with mono-clonality of the T lymphocytes expressing $\gamma\delta$ receptors (those commonly found as intraepithelial lymphocytes). Treatment should be aggressive with systemic steroid therapy and/or immunomodulatory drugs such as azathioprine. Thorough examination for coexistent lymphoma (enteropathy-associated T-cell lymphoma: EATCL) should be made. The prognosis for EATCL or adenocar-cinoma of the small intestine in association with celiac disease is extremely poor with a median survival of 60 days. Presentation is often with perforation. Treatment is by surgery and chemotherapy, although the risk of intestinal perforation in the latter is high.

Patients with celiac disease have a standardized mortality ratio of 2.0. This excess is due to an increase in non-Hodgkin's lymphoma within the first 3 years of diagnosis. It is greatest in those with delayed diagnosis, poor adherence to gluten-free diet and with malabsorption as the presenting symptom. There is an increase in risk of cancer of mouth and pharynx (relative risk = 9.7), esophagus (relative risk = 12.3) and of non-Hodgkin's lymphoma (relative risk = 42.7). The risk returns to that of the general population after taking a gluten-free diet for 5 years.

The outcome in refractory celiac disease is generally poor: in one study of 10 patients with refractory celiac disease, two required total parenteral nutrition, two died and one developed B-cell lymphoma of the ileum.

Family screening

Family members of patients with celiac disease are at increased risk of developing celiac disease (5–18.6% of first-degree relatives have celiac disease) and should be offered screening. Sibs of the proband are at highest risk of developing celiac disease with a lower risk in parents.

IgA EMA has the highest sensitivity and specificity. Total IgA immunoglobulin should be checked and in those with selective IgA deficiency, IgG antigliadin antibodies measured. These have much lower specificity for the disease. Facilities for IgG EMA or transglutaminase antibodies may be available in some centers and show high specificity. In symptomatic relatives, endoscopic distal duodenal biopsies should be obtained as the sensitivity of EMA is only 80%.

Those relatives with positive EMA should have endoscopic distal duodenal biopsies to confirm the diagnosis. Those with positive antibodies but normal histology (or an increase in intraepithelial lymphocytes only) should be considered to have latent disease. They should be kept under follow-up and have a repeat biopsy after 1–2 years or if they become symptomatic. About 50% will develop villous atrophy within 12 months. In a long-term follow-up study, two of 44 relatives with initial negative celiac serology developed celiac disease after 42–102 months, demonstrating the need for repeated testing. Screened celiac patients should be treated in the same way as those presenting with symptomatic disease.

Specialized celiac disease clinics

The BSG recommends that celiac patients are kept under annual review by hospital-based gastroenterologists. In most centers, celiac patients are seen in general gastroenterology clinics.

Specialist clinics have the advantage that most celiac patients will be stable and will not require changes to their therapy. Clinic times are more predictable and prolonged waiting time less common. It is easier to organize dietetic services so that patients can have regular reviews to check not only their compliance with their gluten-free diet, but also the nutritional content of their diet including calcium intake.

Blood tests can be performed 1–2 weeks prior to their clinic visits so that the results are available at clinic and can be discussed. Since most patients will be stable and their management altered little at each visit, these clinics may be led by a clinical nurse specialist in parallel with general gastroenterology clinics. This reduces the need for follow-up in general gastroenterology clinics but permits problems not related to celiac disease to be assessed by medical personnel.

Helpful contacts

The Coeliac Society of the UK, PO Box 220, High Wycombe, Bucks HP11 2HY, UK; Tel: 01494 437273; Fax: 01494 474349; website: www.coeliac.co.uk
Celiac Disease Foundation, 13251 Ventura Boulevard, Suite 1, Studio City, CA 91604–1838 USA; Tel (818) 990-2345; Fax (818) 990-2379; Website: www.celiac.org

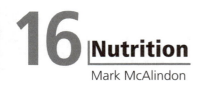

16 |Nutrition

Mark McAlindon

Introduction

Malnutrition (used in this context to describe undernutrition) is common in hospital practice, occurs in all disciplines and has important measurable effects on morbidity and mortality. This chapter will address problems encountered in the outpatient setting: the causes, effects and recognition of malnutrition, nutritional support and its complications in common gastroenterological conditions.

Malnutrition arises because of failure to meet nutritional requirements. This may occur because of inadequate nutritional intake, failure of absorption or a catabolic response in which increased cell metabolism and turnover causes energy demand to exceed supply (see *Figure 16.1*). More than one of these mechanisms may be involved in some patients, such as those with active CD and upper GI malignancy.

Effects of malnutrition

The wide-ranging effects of malnutrition are not always appreciated, and highlight the importance of recognizing and treating undernourished patients.

Early consequences include apathy, depression and anorexia; muscle strength diminishes, which affects ventilatory and cardiac function; impairment of the immune response increases susceptibility to infection, contributes to wound infection and delayed healing. In severely malnourished patients, these combined effects ultimately result in multisystem failure and death (see *Box 16.1*).

All of these factors will affect patient response to pharmacological or surgical treatment, and this has been underscored by numerous studies of many different patient groups. In chronic disorders, nutritional intervention is associated with an improved response to pharmacological treatment, improvement in refractory disease and better quality of

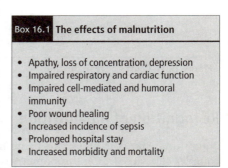

Box 16.1	The effects of malnutrition

- Apathy, loss of concentration, depression
- Impaired respiratory and cardiac function
- Impaired cell-mediated and humoral immunity
- Poor wound healing
- Increased incidence of sepsis
- Prolonged hospital stay
- Increased morbidity and mortality

life. Malnourished surgical patients given nutritional support have fewer septic complications, shorter hospital stay, reduced cost and improved mortality.

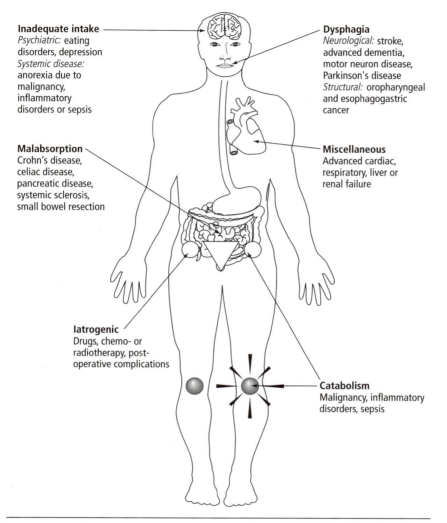

Inadequate intake
Psychiatric: eating disorders, depression
Systemic disease: anorexia due to malignancy, inflammatory disorders or sepsis

Dysphagia
Neurological: stroke, advanced dementia, motor neuron disease, Parkinson's disease
Structural: oropharyngeal and esophagogastric cancer

Malabsorption
Crohn's disease, celiac disease, pancreatic disease, systemic sclerosis, small bowel resection

Miscellaneous
Advanced cardiac, respiratory, liver or renal failure

Iatrogenic
Drugs, chemo- or radiotherapy, post-operative complications

Catabolism
Malignancy, inflammatory disorders, sepsis

Figure 16.1. Causes of malnutrition

Recognition of malnutrition

Nutritional status is measured using many different techniques, including complex clinical scores, anthropometry (a measure of mean arm muscle circumference and triceps skinfold thickness to estimate muscle and fat mass), dynamometry (hand grip strength), biochemical and immunological parameters. Most are research techniques and few are suitable for use as quick outpatient screening tools. However, BMI is a simple measure that should be documented in all patients (*Table 16.1*) and has been used in the development of the Malnutrition Advisory Group screening tool (MAG tool), a measure of malnutrition that provides a score to guide nutritional support (*Figure 16.2*).

Table 16.1. Body mass index (BMI)

(Weight/height^2)		
	< 18.5	Underweight
	18.5–24.9	Normal
	25–30	Overweight
	> 30	Obese

Nutritional support and its complications

The treatment of malnutrition is likely to be one of several interventions in the management of the patient, which may include pharmacological therapy (in inflammatory disorders or sepsis) or surgery. There are several modes of delivering nutritional support, which include oral, enteral tube and parenteral feeding. The gut should be utilized whenever possible as it is more physiological, safer and cheaper.

BMI	Score		% weight loss in last 3–6 months	Score
>20	0		<5%	0
18.5–20	1	**+**	5–10%	1
<18.5	2		>15%	2

Active disease with virtually no intake – score 2

Combined score (BMI + weight loss + active disease with no intake)

0	1	2
Low risk	Medium risk	High risk
No action	Observe	Treat

Figure 16.2. The Malnutrition Advisory Group screening tool

Improving oral intake

The oral intake of many individuals can be improved by expert dietetics assessment and advice. This may be achieved by the use of energy dense meals and the addition of frequent high-calorie, high-protein snacks based on the consumption of real foods from the five food groups (meat and fish, starch foods, milk and dairy products, fats and sugars and fluid). Food fortification by adding milk powder to food or drinks or by using butter, cream and grated cheese in food preparation is another means of increasing calorie intake.

Commercially available sip feeds may also be valuable supplements when used appropriately. They are available as whole protein (polymeric) diets, predigested or 'chemically defined' diets and disease specific diets. Whole protein sip feeds are most commonly used and contain an energy density of 1 kcal ml^{-1} (1.5 kcal ml^{-1} in high-energy feeds) and a nitrogen concentration of 5–7 g l^{-1}. The predigested or 'chemically defined' diets contain synthetic L-amino acids (elemental diet) or oligopeptides as the nitrogen source. They are mainly used in the treatment of active CD, and occasionally in exocrine pancreatic insufficiency or short bowel syndrome. Benefits are largely theoretical as absorption studies have not shown a clear difference between polymeric and elemental diets. Branched-chain amino acid diets have been studied in advanced cirrhosis (see Liver disease, below), but results are not consistent and their role remains unclear.

Appropriate monitoring of supplemented diets is necessary to ensure advice is being followed.

Enteral tube feeding

It is estimated that about 20 000 patients (mainly older adults, but including children) are on home enteral feeding in the UK. Most adults will be fed via a percutaneous endoscopic gastrostomy (PEG), which is considered separately below.

In practice, the commonest indication for outpatient nasoenteral tube feeding in adult gastroenterological practice is the administration of elemental or semi-elemental feeds for the treatment of CD in those who find the diet unpalatable. However, tube feeding may be used in any malnourished patient who cannot attain their requirements because of anorexia, eating or swallowing problems and who have an otherwise intact functioning gut. Contraindications apply almost exclusively to hospitalized patients: paralytic ileus, GI obstruction and major intra-abdominal sepsis.

Most outpatients will be suitable for nasogastric feeding. To minimize the risk of aspiration, nasojejunal (postpyloric) tube feeding should be considered in those with impaired gastric emptying (such as in diabetic gastroparesis), impaired consciousness or in patients without a gag reflex. Some models of nasojejunal tubes are designed to pass spontaneously through the pylorus in subjects with normal gastric emptying. The administration of the prokinetic agents, metoclopramide or erythromycin, may be of benefit in some patients, but endo-scopic or fluoroscopic placement may be required in others.

Complications of enteral feeding mainly relate to the tube or the feed, but metabolic complications also occur (*Table 16.2*). Tube displacement is common, as is blockage. All tubes should be flushed with water after feed administration. Abdominal discomfort, nausea, vomiting and diarrhea may occur, as may regur-gitation and aspiration. GI symptoms may be minimized by using continuous infusion rather than bolus feeding. Side-effects correlate with the osmoles administered per unit time rather than osmoles per unit volume. Most ambulant patients will choose overnight feeding to allow free mobility during the day, but may notice increased nocturnal micturition.

Table 16.2. Tube, feed and metabolic complications of enteral tube feeding

Cause	Complication
Nasoenteral tube	Misplacement
	Dislodgement
	Blockage
Enteral feed	Discomfort, cramps
	Nausea, vomiting
	Regurgitation
	Pulmonary aspiration
	Diarrhea
	Deficiencies of vitamins, minerals, trace elements, essential fatty acids
Metabolic	Hyper/hypokalemia
	Hypo/hyperphosphatemia
	Hyperglycemia
	Hypomagnasemia
	Hypozincemia

Percutaneous endoscopic gastrostomy feeding

PEG feeding is the most common method of giving long-term enteral feeding and should be considered in any patient who requires feeding for more than a few weeks. There is some evidence that PEG feeding improves morbidity and mortality in patients with dysphagic stroke and oropharyngeal malignancies, and these are two of the most common indications in many hospital centers. Other common indications include degenerative neurological disease (advanced dementia, multiple sclerosis, motor neurone and Parkinson's disease) and brain damage due to head injury in which swallowing is impaired. PEG feeding may be considered, however, in any condition in which nutritional intake or absorption is inadequate to meet requirements. Contraindications include bleeding diatheses, gastric or other metastatic cancer, extensive gastric ulceration, intestinal obstruction or ascites. Safe placement is possible in patients with portal hypertension. However, perhaps the commonest and most difficult consider-ation is in deciding whether PEG placement is justified in patients with end-stage disease. Up to a third of patients die within a month or before hospital discharge following PEG placement, and there is evidence to suggest that those with cognitive impairment are in the poorest prognostic group.

PEG placement is a process that involves preassessment and consent, the procedure and aftercare. Most patients are elderly with significant comorbidity. Many neurological patients have impaired ventilatory function and are prone to aspiration. Assessment of fitness for endoscopy and light sedation needs to be done with care. Patients, relatives and carers should be adequately informed about the nature, benefits, risks and alternatives of the procedure in order to provide consent. If the patient does not have capacity to consent, it is lawful to provide treatment without consent for reasons such as temporary unconsciousness, where an emergency situation prevails and if the treatment is in the best interests of the patient and is necessary to save life, ensure improvement or prevent deterioration.

Abdominal examination may reveal evidence of prior surgery, organomegaly or subcutaneous fluid infusions that may make PEG placement more difficult or hazardous. Abnormal clotting should be corrected and the balance of opinion is probably in favor of antibiotic prophylaxis with a broad-spectrum antibiotic (either a cephalosporin or co-amoxyclav).

Although several methods have been described, the 'pull' method of PEG placement is the most commonly used (*Figure 16.3*). The first operator works in a sterile field at the abdominal wall and the second performs the endoscopy and observes the patient's condition. Local anesthetic is instilled into the abdominal wall at a suitable site located by both transillumination (from the tip of the endoscope previously passed into the stomach) and palpation (fingertip depression of the abdominal wall can be seen endoscopically). Failure to achieve both these signs raises the possibility of an interposing organ (colon, small intestine or liver) or much of the stomach being in the chest wall (large hiatus hernia). A cannula is passed into the stomach through which a wire or suture is passed and grasped by an endoscopic snare (see *Figure 16.3*, stages 1 and 2). This is withdrawn *per os* (stage 2), the wire or suture is released by removing the snare and endoscope, and the wire is tied to the PEG (stage 3). The wire, followed by the PEG, is then pulled through the abdominal wall by the first operator (stage 3) who secures it with a fixation device according to the manufacturer's instructions. Some prefer to repeat the endoscopy to ensure correct positioning of the luminal bumper of the PEG, although this may increase risk of aspiration. Others prefer to use the centimeter markers on the tube to alert them to the possibility that the bumper is not abutting the stomach wall and is floating free within the gastric lumen. The fixation device should be loose enough to allow rotation and avoid causing ischemia to the area, but secure enough to prevent significant intraperitoneal leakage. Some models allow the passage of a jejunal feeding tube through the PEG, which can be endoscopically guided into the small bowel (a percutaneous endoscopic gastrojejunostomy) and which may be helpful in patients with impaired gastric emptying or troublesome gastroesophageal reflux. The PEG can be used the day after insertion and the patient should be reviewed to ensure that immediate complications have not occurred.

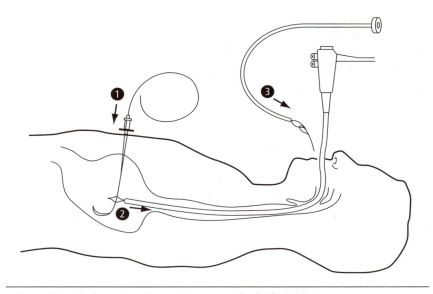

Figure 16.3. The insertion of a percutaneous endoscopic gastrostomy
1. A wire loop is inserted through a cannula into the gastric lumen and secured by a snare placed through the endoscope. 2. Snare and endoscope are withdrawn through the patient's mouth. The wire loop is released and tied to a loop at the end of the PEG. 3. When the wire loop is pulled back through the abdominal wall, the PEG follows until the bumper abuts the gastric wall.

If a suitable insertion site cannot be confidently located, a gastrostomy may be placed under radiological screening after insufflation of the stomach via a nasogastric tube.

PEG complications are common. Minor complications, such as local infections, occur in about 10% of patients. Major complications (aspiration pneumonia, injury to the colon, small bowel or liver) occur in about 5% and there is a PEG-related mortality rate of about 0.5%. The latter figure may be higher if all endoscopy and sedation-related complications are assiduously sought: it has been assumed that the high 1-month-related mortality relates to the underlying disease process, but this may not always be the case.

Most PEG patients are not followed up, although data suggests that longer-term complications are also common. In our hospital center, about a third of patients seek telephone advice about minor complications and over 25% are readmitted. Complications include tube blockage, leakage or inadvertent removal, local sepsis and granulation tissue formation and damage to the fixation device or Y connector (*Figure 16.4*).

If PEGs are pulled out, a replacement gastrostomy may be inserted through the same fistula and a gastric balloon inflated with water to hold the device in place (*Figure 16.5*). The fistula may become difficult to intubate after 6–8 h, although occasionally it may remain patent for longer. Force should not be used

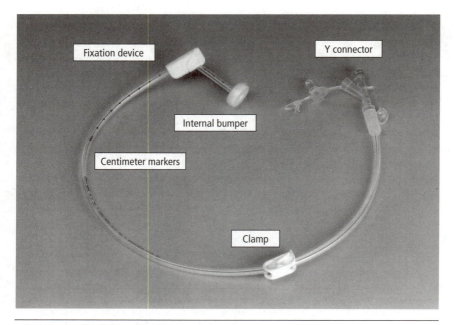

Figure 16.4. A percutaneous endoscopic gastrostomy

in passing anything through the fistula. Correct siting of the replacement gastrostomy can be confirmed using a radiological contrast study via the tube. Patients with sufficient manual dexterity to use a detachable feeding tube may find the low-profile replacement PEGs more cosmetically acceptable (*Figure 16.6*). These are placed percutaneously after the removal of a standard PEG once the gastrocutaneous fistula has formed (6 weeks should allow plenty of time for the fistula to form).

Tube blockage is best avoided by flushing with water after use, including following administration of medications that may damage the tube. Once the fistula has formed, the fixation device should de disconnected and the skin and apparatus washed twice daily with saline and dried. Occasionally blockage, local discomfort, infection, leakage from around the PEG occurs because of 'buried bumper syndrome', in which the bumper becomes embedded in the abdominal wall. If this occurs, the PEG should not be used until this is resolved. Endoscopic release of the bumper has been described using a needle-knife sphincterotome, but some models can be removed percutaneously by traction.

Infection should be treated with appropriate antibiotics after swabs are taken for culture. Excess granulation tissue may be treated by placing an absorbent polyurethane dressing between the fixation device and the skin. Silver nitrate is sometimes used, but produces necrosis and can aggravate local infection or damage adjacent normal skin. Major infection of the abdominal wall is likely to require PEG removal.

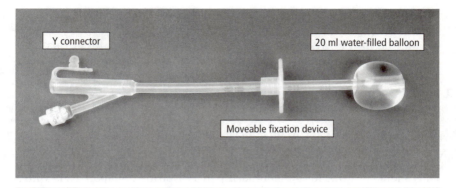

Figure 16.5. Balloon replacement PEG

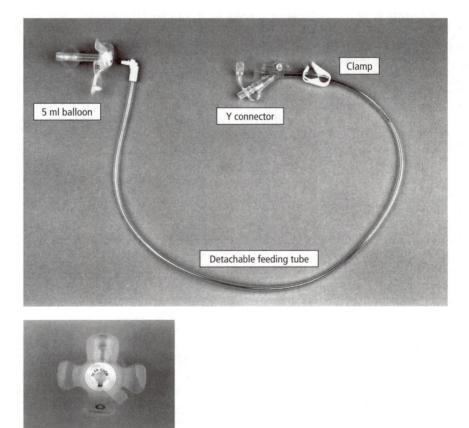

Figure 16.6. Low profile PEG with detachable feeding tube

Nutritional assessment of PEG patients should continue following discharge. The swallowing of some patients may recover sufficiently to allow PEG removal (in up to a fifth of dysphagic stroke patients). As many as 40% of patients continue to have protein-energy malnutrition after discharge and further adjustment to feed and monitoring is necessary.

Home parenteral nutrition

There are about 500 patients on home parenteral nutrition (HPN) in the UK at present. Common indications include CD, ischemic gut, motility disorders, radiation enteritis, congenital bowel disorders, malignancy and AIDS. All patients on HPN should be cared for by a multidisciplinary Nutrition Support Team with a specific interest and expertise in this area. The majority of these patients have frequent hospital contacts. Many are for routine monitoring purposes. However, emergency contacts are common and may occur in centers where the patient is not known. About half of these will relate to the underlying disease process and half to feeding catheter-related complications. The majority of patients know and understand their disease well and are more familiar with line care and its complications than most hospital staff. Any queries about issues relating to HPN patients should be directed to those with an expertise in this area or the Nutrition Support Team responsible for the long-term care of the patient.

Any line handling should be done with meticulous aseptic technique. If the patient is unable to do this, then the line should only be handled by appropriately trained individuals. Poor line care by hospital staff is one of the commonest complaints of HPN patients.

The commonest complications are line blockages, catheter-related septicemia (CRS) or central vein thrombosis. The patient may notice resistance to infusion through the volumetric pump pressure increasing, or that the infusion has simply stopped. This may be due to line kinking, deposition of fibrin, lipid or other debris within the lumen. Occasionally this forms as a sheath on the line tip, impeding withdrawal from the line, but allowing antegrade flow of feed. A chest X-ray should be performed to confirm correct positioning of the line tip. If saline fails to flush the catheter with gentle pressure, an ethanol lock (2 ml of absolute ethanol for 60 min) may free catheters partially occluded after infusion of a lipid mix. Line locks with thrombolytic agents may relieve fibrin occlusion, but ultimately line replacement may be required.

Infection of the catheter may be considered in terms of exit-site infection, tunnel infection or CRS. Exit-site infection can be successfully treated with appropriate antibiotic therapy. It can lead to tunnel infection if the Dacron cuff of the tunneled line is near the exit site and becomes contaminated. Tunnel infection is indicated by pain and redness along the track, and requires catheter removal. Whenever infection is considered, swabs from catheter hub and exit-site and blood from the line should be taken for culture.

CRS is potentially the most serious infective complication and should always be considered in unwell HPN patients. However, HPN patients invariably have complex problems and other causes of sepsis should be considered and actively sought. Bloods should be taken peripherally and from the line for culture. Endoluminal brushes can be used to retrieve samples of the fibrin biofilm lining the catheter for culture, and are particularly useful when blood withdrawal is prevented by a fibrin sheath on the catheter tip. If no other cause of sepsis is evident, feed should be withheld for 24 h until culture results are available. CRS is considered proven if the patient presents with pyrexia and clinically obvious associated tunnel infection, or pyrexia with positive blood or swab cultures and resolution after appropriate therapy (antibiotics or removal of line). Probable CRS is defined as pyrexia with no other obvious source of infection and resolution after appropriate therapy when blood and swab cultures are not taken or results are inconclusive. CRS is considered possible when pyrexia occurs in the presence of a possible alternative source of infection without supporting blood culture evidence of CRS, but in which pyrexia resolves after antibiotic therapy or removal of the line.

Staphylococcus epidermis and *S. aureus* are the commonest infections. Yeast infections are relatively common and Gram-negative organisms are implicated in a small minority of cases. CRS due to *S. aureus* or *Candida albicans* respond poorly to antimicrobial therapy and is likely to require removal of the line. Failure to respond to 48 h of treatment may also indicate a need to remove the line.

Teicoplanin has bacterial activity against Gram-positive bacteria, particularly *S. aureus,* and is a commonly used first-line treatment of suspected CRS until sensitivities are available. Teicoplanin locks are left in the line between infusions and withdrawn immediately before the next infusion is given. Blood cultures should be taken through the catheter at least 12–24 h after the last infusion to confirm successful treatment. The line should not be used during treatment.

Central vein thrombosis should be suspected in any HPN patient presenting with swelling of the limb, face or neck. There may be dilated collateral blood vessels on the chest. Doppler scanning or upper limb venography should be arranged urgently, anticoagulation treatment commenced and the line removed.

Malnutrition and nutritional support in gastroenterology

Inflammatory bowel disease

Malnutrition affects 30–50% of patients requiring admission for treatment of IBD. Two-thirds of patients with active CD and up to half of those with active UC have weight loss. Growth retardation and delayed puberty are well-recognized phenomena in children adolescents with CD. Deficiencies of vitamins and trace elements are described, particularly in CD. The development of malnutrition is multifactorial in origin. Patients may be anorexic or restricting intake to control symptoms. Drugs (steroids, sulfasalazine and cholestyramine) interfere with vitamin absorption and turnover of trace elements. Malabsorption occurs because of small bowel mucosal injury and inflamed gut mucosa loses protein, blood, electrolytes, minerals and trace elements. In addition to these losses, there may be an increased nutritional requirement because of sepsis and increased cell turnover.

Nutritional support not only improves nutritional parameters, but also improves outcome in refractory CD, so should be considered as an essential part of the management of patients. Oral nutritional support (with standard diet or whole protein sip feed supplements) seems to be no less effective than parenteral nutrition, so should be used in the presence of an intact gut. Elemental or semi-elemental diet (oligopeptide) diets are widely used in the treatment of active CD. They are probably slightly less effective but have fewer adverse effects than steroids as primary therapy. Many physicians use them as first-line treatment, particularly in patients at risk of steroid side-effects or in whom weight loss is a significant feature.

Nutritional support in UC has not been studied in the same detail as in CD, but the same principles should apply. Enteral feeding is well tolerated in acute UC and, indeed, is probably safer and as effective as parenteral nutrition in severe disease.

Liver disease

Many factors contribute to the widespread prevalence of malnutrition in advanced chronic liver disease. Severe malnutrition is associated with increased mortality in patients with alcoholic hepatitis, cirrhosis and after liver transplantation. Intake may be inadequate because of anorexia, dietary restriction and adverse effects of drugs. In alcohol abuse, alcohol forms the major contributor to daily calorie consumption at the expense of protein, fat and carbohydrate. Reduced choleresis causes malabsorption of fat and fat-soluble vitamins, and both alcohol and liver dysfunction may impair the conversion of water-soluble vitamins to their active components. Paracentesis, bleeding and sepsis cause nutrient loss and protein-calorie demand is increased.

Malnourished outpatients with alcoholic cirrhosis may have fewer infective complications and hospital admissions if given a standard supplemented diet. Following the identification of low levels of branched-chain and high levels of aromatic amino acids (which are neurotransmitter precursors) in liver disease, considerable interest has been shown in the use of diets supplemented with branched-chain amino acids in alcoholic hepatitis and hepatic encaphalopathy. However, only a minority of studies show a benefit in favor of branched-chain amino acids, and routine use cannot be recommended at present. What these and other studies do suggest is that severely ill, malnourished patients in negative nitrogen balance have a high mortality rate and may benefit from aggressive nutritional support. There is little evidence that protein restriction is necessary in encephalopathy and some evidence that moderate amounts of protein may improve recovery.

Short bowel syndrome

The small intestine is between 3 and 8 m in length. Given this variability, it is important to know the residual length of small bowel, rather than the amount resected at surgery. The common clinical situations are either that the patient has a jejunostomy following extensive small bowel and colonic resection, or a jejuno-colonic anastomosis following a small bowel resection.

Most patients with 50 cm or more of the small intestine anastomosed to some residual colon, or with 100 cm or more of small bowel ending in a jejunostomy will manage without resource to long-term intravenous fluids or nutrition. This may not be the case if the residual bowel functions poorly, as may occur in CD, systemic sclerosis or radiation injury. Some patients with less extensive resections may still require oral or enteral supplements.

Jejunostomy patients may lose between 2 and 8 l of fluid per day, composed of gastric and pancreaticobiliary secretions and oral intake. Jejunal mucosa is highly permeable, so hypotonic fluids taken by mouth tend to cause flux of sodium down the concentration gradient into the jejunal lumen, resulting in salt and water loss. Hypotonic fluid should therefore be restricted to less than 500 ml daily. The normal sodium concentration at the duodenal–jejunal flexure is about 90 mmol. Sodium absorption can only occur against a small concentration gradient and is coupled to glucose absorption and that of some amino acids. A glucose–saline solution with a sodium concentrate of 90–120 mmol (the WHO cholera solution without potassium chloride contains 90 mmol sodium) can be given, although not all find this sufficiently palatable for long-term consumption. High doses of loperamide (up to 16 mg daily) may be needed as normal enterohepatic recirculation is disrupted and codeine phosphate may provide some additional benefit. PPIs and octreotide are commonly used as antisecretory agents. Magnesium losses are high and supplements may be required.

The colon has a large capacity to absorb salt and water, so fluid loss does not present the same problem in patients with jejunocolic anastomoses as in those with a jejunostomy. However, loss of the major nutrient absorptive surface means that they are prone to malnutrition and require high-energy diets. The diet should be high in carbohydrate, as polysaccharides are fermented in the colon and absorbed as short-chain fatty acids, a rich energy source. Unabsorbed free fatty acids may contribute to diarrhea by interfering with salt and water absorption and affecting colonic transit, so some restriction of dietary fat is necessary. Medium-chain triglycerides provide energy and can be absorbed in the colon. Abnormal colonization of the residual small bowel by microbes containing D-lactate dehydrogenase may lead to D-lactic (as opposed to the commonly measured L(+) lactate isomer) acidosis during fermentation of a carbohydrate load. Patients present with ataxia, blurred vision, ophthalmoplegia and nystagmus and have a metabolic acidosis with a large anion gap. Treatment is with broad-spectrum antibiotics, thiamine and a diet high in polysaccharides and low in mono- and oligosaccharides.

Two factors contribute to excessive oxalate absorption in patients with a jejunocolic anastomosis: free fatty acids preferentially bind calcium, thus releasing oxalate for absorption, and unabsorbed bile salts enhance colonic permeability to oxalate. Therefore, patients are at considerable risk of oxalate renal stones and dietary oxalate should be restricted. Foods rich in oxalate include tea, rhubarb and spinach.

Further reading

Cabré, E. and Gassull, M.A. (1995) Nutritional support in liver disease. *Eur. J. Gastroenterol. Hepatol.* **7**: 528–532.

Geerling, B.J., Stockbrügger, R.W. and Brummer, R.-J.M. (1999) Nutrition and inflammatory bowel disease. *Scand. J. Gastroenterol.* **34** (Suppl. 230): 95–105.

González-Huix, F., Fernández-Bañares, F., Esteve-Comas, M., *et al.* (1993). Enteral versus parenteral nutrition as adjunct therapy in acute ulcerative colitis. *Am. J. Gastroenterol.* **88**: 227–232.

Greenberg, G.R., Fleming, C.R., Jeejeebhoy, K.N., Rosenberg, I.H., Sales, D. and Tremaine, W.J. (1988) Controlled trial of bowel rest and nutrition support in the management of Crohn's disease. *Gut* **29**: 1309–1315.

Griffiths, A.M., Ohlsson, A., Sherman, P.M. and Sutherland, L.R. (1995) Meta-analysis of enteral nutrition as a primary treatment of active Crohn's disease. *Gastroenterology* **108**: 1056–1067.

Morgan, B.J., Taylor, M.B. and Johnson, C.D. (1990) Percutaneous endoscopic gastrostomy. *Br. J. Surg.* **77**: 858–862.

Müller, M.J. (1995) Malnutrition in cirrhosis. *J. Hepatol.* **23** (Suppl. 1): 31–35.

Nightingale, J.M.D. (1995) Nutritional support in gastroenterology: the short bowel syndrome. *Eur. J. Gastroenterol. Hepatol.* **7**: 514–520.

Pennington, C.R., Fawcett, H., Macfie, J., McWhirter, J., Sizer, T. and Whitney, S. (1996) Current perspectives on parenteral nutrition in adults. British Association for Parenteral and Enteral Nutrition (BAPEN) Redditch, UK.

Sanders, D.S., Carter, M.J., D'Silva, J., James, G., Bolton, R.P. and Bardhan, K.D. (2000) Survival analysis in percutaneous endoscopic gastrostomy: a worse outcome in patients with dementia. *Am. J. Gastroenterol.* **95**: 1472–1475.

Sanders, D.S., Carter, M.J., D'Silva, J.D., McAlindon, M.E., Willemse, P.J. and Bardhan, K.D. (2001) Percutaneous endoscopic gastrostomy: a prospective analysis of hospital support required and complications following discharge to the community. *Eur. J. Clin. Nutr.* **55**: 610–614.

Seymour, C.A. and Whelan, K. (1999) Dietary management of hepatic encephalopathy. *Br. Med. J.* **318**: 1364–1365.

17 | Developing a Successful Gastrointestinal Service

Harry Dalton, Hyder Hussaini and Iain Murray

Teamwork

Delivering any successful service depends on developing a properly functioning team. For a team to function effectively, each team member must be able to respect and trust all the others. Furthermore, the team must appreciate that all the members have differing roles, responsibilities and abilities. Each member has an important role to play in the effective delivery of the service. This applies as much to the ward cleaners as it does to the consultant staff.

The members of our GI team are shown in *Table 17.1*. As can be seen, there are a very large number of individuals in the team with diverse backgrounds, skills and personalities. How have we managed to mold them into an effective team?

Table 17.1. Members of the gastrointestinal (GI) team

Consultant gastroenterologists
Consultant GI surgeons
Consultant GI radiologists
Consultant GI pathologists
Consultant GI oncologists
Junior medical staff
Palliative care physicians
Nursing staff
Ward
Outpatients
Endoscopy
Research fellow
Research nurse
Secretaries
Reception staff (Endoscopy Unit and Outpatient Department)
Radiographers
Porters
Cleaners

Building an effective team

Choosing individuals with appropriate team-working skills

An effective team requires individuals with differing team-working skills: leaders, innovators, completers–finishers, workers and organizers. For a team to function successfully, it is essential that the individual attributes of the team are balanced. For example, a dysfunctional group would results if all members of the team were strong on leadership skills.

Team identity

It is important that the individuals that make up the team feel part of the team. This can be achieved in a number of ways. The whole team must meet on a regular basis. In our institution, we have 2-monthly GI unit meetings at which progress is assessed, problems addressed and new ideas discussed. All members of the team are invited.

Other approaches we have used include displaying a photograph of members of the team at the entrance of the unit and employing a unit letterhead, which includes physicians, surgeons, radiologists, histopathologists and oncologists.

We regularly teach our undergraduate students as a team – this has been a very useful way to ensure that the student teaching is never canceled, but has also been an invaluable team-building exercise as we have developed our teaching skills together (see Chapter 19).

In the future, we are planning to learn advanced cardiac life support as a multidisciplinary team. All members of staff will be invited, from the most junior nursing student to the most senior consultant. This will not only be an important way of refreshing our cardiopulmonary resuscitation skills but should help consolidate individuals in the team.

Developing a patient-centered approach

Being ill is not a pleasant experience. We feel that it is our responsibility to make a patient's illness as bearable as possible. This implies not only top-quality evidence-based care but also delivery of care in a manner and environment that we would wish for our family or ourselves.

We have, therefore, paid considerable attention to the patient environment. The corridor in our GI unit has recently been decorated by local artists. It is extraordinarily eye-catching and we have had universal praise from both patients and staff. The idea of the corridor was to grab the patients' attention, even if only for a moment, to deflect their minds from worry over the reason they were in hospital (e.g. a colonoscopy).

Patients on our ward often feel lonely and isolated and are often many miles from home. We have recently commissioned a series of photographs of scenes from Cornwall, which are now on the walls of our unit. This makes the ward look more pleasant, and the patients feel at home (*Figure 17.1*).

Patients with GI problems attend our unit from a very wide geographical area. It is not uncommon for patients to travel 40 miles to come to clinic. Consider what happens to a patient who has been referred with abdominal pain. The GP sends the referral letter. The patient is seen in the outpatient department. Some blood tests are performed and an upper GI endoscopy and abdominal

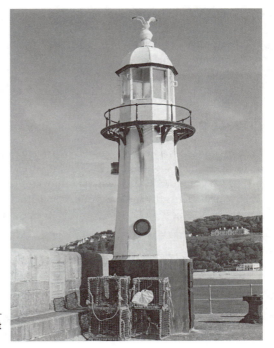

Figure 17.1. Gastrointestinal unit photograph: St. Ives.

ultrasound scan are requested. The diagnosis turns out to be an HP-positive duodenal ulcer. Treatment is started and the patient's progress is reviewed 8 weeks later in clinic. The patient is now better and discharged. This patient therefore attended on four occasions and traveled a total distance of 320 miles.

We now manage such patients using a one-stop approach (see Chapter 1). Employing the one-stop approach to the above scenario would have resulted in the patient traveling 80 miles for a single visit. We have successfully introduced a similar one-stop approach in several other areas including iron deficiency anemia, rectal bleeding and jaundice and are developing a similar service for patients with dysphagia (see Chapters 2, 3, 4 and 5).

Another factor that influences the quality of patient care is the physical layout of the GI unit. In our unit the endoscopy suite, the GI medical and surgical wards, the radiology department and the unit's secretarial offices are all situated in very close proximity on the same floor. This enhances patient care by improving working relationships within the team. In an ideal world, the GI outpatient facility would also be situated within the same area.

Developing the service

Developing any service within the cash-strapped NHS is nearly always a challenge and often disheartening. We have achieved a great deal in a very short space of time by adopting the following approach:

- Develop a good working relationship with the hospital management.
- Project the team as proactive and dynamic.
- Always have a business plan ready.
- Innovate as much as possible.
- Publicize successful innovations.
- Develop new ways of generating income (see later)

Private practice

Private practice is usually discussed in private. It is an area worthy of discussion, as by applying a few basic principles, it is relatively straightforward to build a thriving private practice. The most important thing about private medicine is to treat your patients the same as your NHS patients. The only difference is that the patient is paying for your time and you therefore have the luxury of spending more time with each patient.

There are three attributes a gastroenterologist requires to build a successful private practice. These are the 'three As': ability, availability, affability.

These characteristics speak for themselves.

When starting a private practice it is necessary to register with the insurance companies, arrange for admitting rights to the local private hospital and arrange a private secretary, book-keeper and accountant. Most private hospitals have endoscopic facilities, although these can be of variable quality. Usually, the private hospital charges the consultant for room-time for outpatient clinics, but there is no charge to the consultant for using the endoscopic facilities. This is billed to the insurance company or patient, if uninsured.

Private practice can be a major bone of contention. Jealousy and competition between consultants over private practice is frequently the source of major disagreements between senior members of the GI team. When this happens, the team may cease to function effectively. We have taken the radical approach that the consultants who do private practice share the workload and income. This has numerous benefits. There is no jealousy/competition, it promotes effective team-working, provides improved patient care, and income continues when on holiday or when sick. However, this only works because the individuals concerned respect and trust each other both professionally and personally.

Over the last 18 months, we have been performing our private endoscopic procedures in a vacant slot in the endoscopy unit in the NHS GI unit. This is a fairly major departure from normal practice in our hospital where, in the past, little or no private medicine has been performed. This was achieved by developing a business plan, which was presented to the Trust Board. The business plan demonstrated a clear financial benefit to the hospital from hospital fees, which would normally have gone to the private hospital. Furthermore, extra staff were appointed, including a research fellow, research nurse, research/private secretary and an additional endoscopy nurse. Whilst some of these individuals spend some of their time helping to run the private endoscopy slot, the rest of their working time is spent on NHS activities. This was well received by the Trust Board.

It was agreed by the Gastrointestinal Unit staff and the Trust Board that the private endoscopy initiative would not impinge on NHS work in any way whatsoever. On the contrary, running the private list has had several major benefits for our NHS patients. It also removes patients from the NHS waiting list.

The private endoscopy list is run on a vacant morning slot, where normally no NHS funding is available to provide endoscopy. Performing the private procedures therefore allows us to fully staff the unit during the whole morning. When the private procedures are completed, NHS patients requiring emergency endoscopy are seen. This usually amounts to two or three NHS patients per morning. These patients would otherwise have had to wait until the following morning for their endoscopies.

The financial arrangements for the running of the private endoscopy initiative are shown in *Table 17.2*. All hospital profits are ring-fenced for use in developing the GI unit. This has generated an annual income of approximately £150 000 and allowed us to introduce EUS and appoint a research fellow, research nurse and research secretary. It should be noted that these arrangements have not adversely affected the private income of the gastroenterologists involved with the scheme.

Table 17.2. The private patient initiative: finance

Procedure	Hospital charge (early 2002)
EGD	£210
Flexible sigmoidoscopy	£210
Colonoscopy	£360
Therapeutic ERCP	£1030

EGD, esophagogastroduodenoscopy; ERCP, endoscopic retrograde cholangiopancreatography. The cost of running an average list (consumables) is approximately £135; the cost per patient (consumables) for performing ERCP is approximately £530.

Research

In a busy clinical gastroenterological practice, it is difficult to find the time to have active research interests. It is even more difficult to obtain funding. Identifying a source of money generated locally (private patient initiative, see above) has allowed us to appoint several research staff, including a full-time research fellow. This has enabled us to pursue and develop our interests in IBD, HCV and medical education.

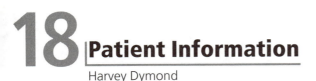

Patient Information

Harvey Dymond

Introduction

There are numerous ways in which patients gain information about their diagnosis, treatment or impending hospital procedures. These include word-of-mouth, glossy leaflets and in recent years the Internet. The quality of information that can be obtained from these sources is variable. The imparting of information is a key component in many aspects of patient care not least within the consent process. To this end, novel approaches can be employed to more effectively achieve informed consent. Other innovative approaches such as a nurse-counselor improves the quality of the overall service available to patients as well as in the way information is given to them.

Leaflets

Leaflets are one of the more traditional methods of imparting information to patients. Over the years, many have been produced of variable quality. While some are undoubtedly well researched and thoughtfully prepared, others are less helpful and poorly thought out. Leaflets have a tendency either not to be read, or to be picked up and then forgotten about.

Careful thought and targeting is required if the maximum benefit is to be derived from the production of a leaflet. Some important issues need to be considered when designing a leaflet:

- Is the main message accessible?
- Is compliance and patient satisfaction improved?
- Does the design and content account for the educational level and the reading and comprehension abilities of the target audience?

Having produced a leaflet, or when judging the suitability of those produced by others, four basic questions need to be satisfied:

- Is the information of use to patients?
- Can they understand and recall it?
- Does it increase compliance?
- Are patients satisfied with the content?

While much has been written about the readability of leaflets there is far less work on their ability to get their particular message across. A well-produced leaflet has an important role to play in supplementing and reinforcing information given verbally. Such a leaflet needs to contain good-quality evidence-based information that is clearly communicated; and needs to involve patients as well as healthcare professionals in the development and evaluation stages.

Patient information center

It is important that people have accurate and relevant written information that they can take away with them for future reference. To maintain such a resource effectively can present staff with difficulties. A central point where a library of appropriate leaflets and other information can be maintained is one such solution to the problem. A resource center maintained by people with librarian-type skills offers an opportunity to develop an integrated information resource that goes beyond traditional methods of distributing information. Having a system in place where patients (and/or their relatives) can either visit of their own volition or be referred to is better than an informal and possibly haphazard method of giving leaflets on an *ad hoc* basis with some people receiving the information and others not. The main advantages of such a center are summarized in *Box 18.1*.

Patient information centers do have some disadvantages that need to be recognized and understood. They are likely to be available during office hours only and not available at weekends or in the evening if a clinic overruns. The gastro-enterology team may have little control over what gastro-enterology information is to be stocked. In a large hospital, the center may not be located geographically close to the gastroenterology unit or outpatient clinic. Finally, the staff employed may not have specialist gastro-enterology knowledge or experience.

> **Box 18.1 Main advantages of a patient information center**
>
> - Greater variety of up-to-date information than would otherwise be possible on a ward or endoscopy unit
> - Utilization of different modalities of delivering information, e.g. video or computer
> - Prevents duplication
> - Staff in the information center develop experience and expertise in obtaining and then disseminating this type of information
> - Cost effective – information available from across all specialties
> - Can be visited by patients at times other than when visiting for clinical purposes
> - Gastroenterology staff time not spent managing information resources

We have found that the patient information center at our institution is an invaluable adjunct to patient care. It is called the 'Information Link' and was established in 1994. It provides a centralized information and resource point for an 850-bedded district general hospital serving a population of 385 000 people. The center receives on average 350 inquiries a month, of which approximately 10% of these are gastroenterology related. The hospital's general office is located within the center maximizing the facilities patients, visitors and staff can access from one location.

The center not only provides information in the form of traditional leaflets and other printed material, but also provides computer facilities, videos and a wealth of reference material. They also encourage patient groups to hold exhibitions within the center. A recent exhibitor was the local NACC group.

Further developments could include enabling patients to access the Internet from the resource center or for the center to develop its own Internet site so patients can access or order information online.

Taking the concept a stage further could involve establishing links with local university medical and nursing schools. Students would become involved in the patient information center as part of a communications module. This would have benefits for both patients and students.

For patients, it would give them the opportunity to speak to people with a greater medical knowledge than would otherwise be available in the center and without the time constraints of a standard outpatient consultation. This approach could be of equal benefit to not only the anxious or distressed patient who may need that additional time to work things through, but also the patient who wants to know everything. For students, it would provide invaluable experience in talking to and teaching patients as well as enabling them to focus on their communication skills in general.

Nurse-counselor

The Nurse-counselor role differs from the traditional specialist nurse role in that a nurse with developed counseling skills, gained through both specialist training and experience, is utilized. This individual not only provides counseling and support but also has the clinical experience necessary to provide relevant information, education and advice to patients and their families. From the counseling perspective it is more than just having someone to talk to but rather someone who can provide therapeutic counseling. This encourages patients to explore the anxieties, feelings and problems that are experienced when trying to live with a chronic disease.

There are a number of facets to such a role: firstly, in the outpatients department, endoscopy unit and ward when the counselor either participates or is available for patients when they are given emotionally traumatic information such as a diagnosis of malignant disease. Their role in these circumstances is to reinforce explanations about disease management and to discuss implications with individuals. In this way, patient concerns can be supported and follow-up negotiated. Secondly, additional specialist support to individuals who have complex problems and are in need of more specific psychological support. Finally, there is the group of people who are referred directly, following psychological assessment, for therapeutic counseling sessions.

In the field of IBD, such a service is not only highly valued by patients but also gives them the opportunity to discuss wide-ranging issues. These include experiences such as the anxiety, depression and anger caused by the effects of their illness, which cannot be explored effectively during a standard medical consultation.

Internet

The Internet is a potential source of information on a scale previously unavailable to patients. Patients who have access to the Internet are often better informed than previous generations, a trend which is certain to increase as more people go online.

However, with the explosion of health-related Internet sites, there are questions over their potential disadvantages to patients. The accuracy and legitimacy of some of the information and advice given by some sites can be dubious if not potentially dangerous. New sites seem to appear daily, and while some existing sites are constantly being modified and updated, others are rarely modified and may contain out-of-date information or advice. Some information may give people unrealistic expectations or make them reject other legitimate and proven techniques that would be of benefit to them. Consequently, patients (and staff) need to be cautioned about the pitfalls of taking such information at face value.

A quality standard (e.g. a kite mark) given to a site that meets certain quality criteria would be a way forward in highlighting the quality and legitimacy of the information contained within a site. Such criteria are likely to include information that accords with the available evidence and been presented in a useful and an acceptable form. However, to undertake such an enterprise requires no small effort and resources. Only a small proportion of sites could ever be validated in such a way or indeed allow themselves to be subjected to such a validation process.

However, many people are experienced at using the Internet and would expect to obtain the information they need from several sources. By applying critical thinking, patients are often able to distinguish the relevant and reliable information from the more dubious.

Using the following steps as a guide, the content of online information can, to a degree, be evaluated:

- Do not judge a website by its appearance. While a professional-looking site may well contain more accurate information then a poorly organized one, it may also just be a slick marketing ploy for a quack health remedy
- Try to find out who is behind the information. Be very skeptical if the author or creator is not identified
- Try to determine why the information has been posted. Individuals or groups may have their own agenda that could be either hidden or explicit
- Check the date of information. Some sites are frequently updated but others may have been forgotten by their authors and contain out-of-date and inaccurate information
- Try to verify the same information elsewhere. This is especially important if it is contrary to your current knowledge of a subject
- Try to find out how others feel about the reliability of the site. Evaluations of sites are offered by a number of review guides

It is important to remember that many people do not have Internet access and therefore have to rely on more traditional sources of information.

Informed consent

It is imperative that when patients are giving their consent to any invasive procedure they are to undergo they do so from an informed and autonomous perspective. To this end a brief verbal explanation just before the procedure and the signing of a consent form does not suffice. A more robust mechanism is required whereby patients are given more detailed information, well before their procedure, giving them time to digest it and formulate any questions they may have for the day of the procedure.

There are a number of ways in which this requirement could be met. A common approach is to send out information leaflets pre-procedure. A novel solution is to have the consent form incorporated into an information leaflet (see *Figure 18.1a–c*) so as to link the information-giving process with the consent process. This method, as well as providing information about what to expect before, during and after the procedure, gives patients an insight into the consent process itself before they are actually required to give consent. It insures all patients receive, at the very least, a minimum acceptable level of information. The consent form section of the leaflet can be devised in such a way that it is 'condition-specific' and thus have greater relevance to the procedure to be undergone and in itself provide a reinforcement of the information given in the preceding leaflet.

Such a tool serves two purposes for the staff. It provides an effective way of imparting initial information to patients, which can then be built upon when they attend hospital. Secondly, because the consent form is an integral part of the information leaflet it provides a method of demonstrating the quality and quantity of information a patient has received prior to their procedure.

Giving or posting the combined leaflet some days before attendance for the procedure gives patients time to read it several times so maximizing the opportunity for the information contained within it to be absorbed. Such a process also provides patients with the time to formulate any questions the may have.

For such a scenario to be effective, the consent process itself becomes a four-stage process:

1. A medical practitioner (hospital doctor or GP) identifies the need and appropriateness of an endoscopic procedure and ideally explains the procedure and why it is required.
2. The patient receives the information in the form of a combined leaflet/consent form.
3. The nursing staff on the ward or endoscopy unit (or both) reinforces the information. The patient should then be in a position to complete his/her section of the consent form.
4. Prior to the procedure, the endoscopist satisfies him/herself that the patient understands the risks, benefits and alternatives. The endoscopist then completes his/her section of the consent form.

Royal Cornwall Hospitals **NHS**
NHS Trust

ERCP

What is an ERCP?

ERCP stands for Endoscopic Retrograde Cholangio-Pancreatography. This procedure allows the endoscopist to take detailed X-rays of your pancreas and bile ducts. A long flexible tube (endoscope) is passed through your mouth, gullet (oesophagus), and stomach into the upper part of your small intestine (duodenum). Once the endoscope is in position, special dye is injected down the endoscope, so that the pancreas and bile ducts can be seen on X-ray film.

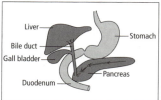

Why do I need an ERCP?

ERCP is used to diagnose and treat disorders of the bile ducts and pancreas. This test is usually performed when patients are jaundiced, following pancreatitis and in certain patients with gallstones prior to an operation to remove the gallbladder (cholecystectomy).

ERCP is much safer than the old fashioned alternative which was an operation to explore the bile ducts or pancreas.

What treatment can be done during an ERCP?

Sphincterotomy: If the X-ray shows a gallstone, which has slipped down into the bile duct, the endoscopist will enlarge the opening of the duct with an electrically heated wire called a diathermy. Any stones are collected by the endoscopist or are left to pass into the intestine.

Stenting: If the X-ray shows a narrowing of the bile duct, the endoscopist may need to place a short plastic bypass tube (stent) in the duct. This allows the bile to drain into the bowel again. The stent may be left in permanently, although it may be necessary to replace it later if it becomes blocked. You will not be aware of the tube inside you.

What do I need to do to prepare for the test?

You should have nothing to eat or drink for at least 6 hours (and preferably overnight) before the ERCP, although you can drink a small cup of water if you're very thirsty. Regular prescription medication can be taken.

What will happen?

Before the test you will be asked to undress, put on a hospital gown and remove any glasses or dentures. An endoscopist and/or nurse will explain the procedure to you. Please make sure you inform the endoscopist if you:

- have any heart or lung problems, have diabetes or other medical problems
- have any allergies
- have an artificial heart valve or have suffered from an infected heart valve (endocarditis)
- are taking medicines to thin your blood e.g. warfarin/aspirin

The endoscopist will insert a small plastic needle (cannula) into your arm, through which we can give you any necessary medication. We will take you on a bed to the X-ray department, where the endoscopist will answer any further questions or concerns that you have about the test.

You will be asked to lie comfortably on your left side with your left arm behind your back so that we can roll you onto your stomach once the procedure is underway. A sedative injection will be given to make you sleepy. You should not remember anything of the test. The endoscope is then passed through your mouth into your throat. The tube will not cause you any pain, and will not interfere with your breathing. A mouth guard will protect your teeth. The endoscope is

Figure 18.1. Patient information sheet/consent form for endoscopic retrograde cholangiopancreatography (ERCP). (a) Page 1; (b) page 2; (c) page 3 – this page is detachable and once signed is placed in the patient's notes.

(b)

passed through the stomach into the upper intestine and the examination is carried out. The test itself lasts between 15-60 minutes. Usually you will stay in hospital overnight.

What happens after an ERCP?

We will keep you under observation until the effects of the sedation have worn off; your stay in hospital may be extended for a few days if further checks or treatment is necessary. The endoscopist will discuss the results of the ERCP with you before you leave hospital.

What are the common risks of ERCP?

There may be a slight risk to crowned teeth or dental bridgework, and you should tell the endoscopist if you have either of these.

Other risks vary with the reasons we did the test, what was found, the treatment carried out (if any) and other existing medical problems. In general, endoscopy can result in complications, such as reactions to medication, perforation of the intestine, and bleeding.

Complications after a diagnostic ERCP (no treatment carried out) are less than after therapeutic ERCP (where treatment is carried out), but include:

- 1-2% risk of pancreatitis (inflammation of the pancreas)
- allergic reactions to the dye used in taking an X-ray (rare)
- infection of the bile duct called cholangitis (rare)

Therapeutic ERCP (treatment for stones or blockage of the bile duct) is recommended, because it is simpler and safer than standard surgical operations. However, you should realise that they are not always successful, and possible complications can arise including:

- 5% risk of pancreatitis (inflammation of the pancreas)
- 2% risk of bleeding from the sphincterotomy site
- 1% risk of infection of the bile duct (cholangitis)
- 0.3% risk of perforation of the intestine
- 0.4% risk related mortality rate

Pancreatitis can be a severe (1:14 cases) potentially life threatening condition. The risk of pancreatitis in an individual patient may be greater depending on the indications for ERCP. If you have concerns regarding your risk, this should be discussed with the doctor prior to ERCP.

These complications are rare, but may require urgent treatment, and even an operation. Be sure to inform us if you have any pain, fever or vomiting during the 24 hours after your ERCP.

Many months after an ERCP, bile duct stents can become blocked with debris. This will result in the jaundice coming back, and you may also have fevers and chills. If this happens, you should inform your GP. You will need antibiotics, and a possible change of stent.

Final points

Don't worry if you do not remember all you have read, as you will have plenty of opportunity to discuss the test and your condition with the medical and nursing staff.

If you have any queries at all please ask or phone the Endoscopy Unit on:

We want to make sure that you are completely comfortable about the procedure

---

(c)

Endoscopy Consent Form

Please complete the following:

Patient's surname ....
First name ....   Patient's label
Date of birth ....
Address ....
....

I have read and understood the information sheet opposite. I therefore give informed consent to have an:

ERCP

I understand that:

- a trained endoscopist will perform the procedure
- additional procedures may need to be performed if clinically indicated
- I can decide not to undergo this procedure
- there is a risk of damage to the bile duct, cholangitis (infection in the bile duct) or pancreatitis (inflammation of the pancreas)
- if a sphincterotomy is necessary then the risk of haemorrhage or perforation is increased
- if a stent is inserted through an area of narrowing in the bile duct or pancreas to relieve jaundice, again cholangitis or pancreatitis may occasionally occur
- the stent may need to be replaced from time to time
- there is a slight risk to crowned teeth or dental bridgework.

Patient's signature: .... **Date:** ....

(only sign if you have no additional questions regarding your ERCP)

Endoscopist's declaration

I declare that the patient named above understands the:

- nature
- alternatives
- indications
- common complications

of this endoscopic procedure and thus gives informed consent.

Additional comments (eg. if patient is unable to give consent)

Endoscopist's signature: .... **Date:** ....

This process gives patients the opportunity to assimilate the information they are given, and make an informed decision.

Level of information

The issues discussed so far concern the modalities for imparting information as opposed to the level of information an individual requires. Individual people need information to be presented at different levels and in different formats. While there has been debate about the level at which written information should be pitched – usually based on average reading ages or educational attainment – there is less clarity about dealing with people face-to-face. At this level, it is not so easy for healthcare practitioners to determine the level of information a patient needs. While this may not be a simple issue to resolve it must nevertheless be borne in mind.

Summary

Leaflets are a traditional method of providing information to patients. To be of maximum benefit they need to be well devised and targeted appropriately. When managed in a coordinated manner, patient information centers can achieve this objective by providing a library of up-to-date accessible information. They also provide the potential to develop other services, which can be integrated into the center.

The nurse-counselor role gives patients access to an experienced healthcare professional, who not only is a source of practical information and support but can also provide therapeutic counseling for those in need of it.

The consent process is one that in which the receiving and retention of accurate information is essential. Incorporating the consent form into an information leaflet offers the opportunity to improve the information given and insure that everyone receives consistent information in a way that allows them to re-read it as much and whenever necessary.

The Internet offers a huge potential source of information but some of it can be of dubious quality and both patients and healthcare professionals need to be aware of this. Kite-marking of 'approved' sites could provide a way forward, although this is a complex issue and only a relatively small proportion of sites are ever likely to participate in such a scheme.

Acknowledgment

We thank Dr S.H. Hussaini and the Royal Cornwall Hospitals (NHS) Trust for the use of the ERCP combined information sheet and consent form in this chapter.

Further reading

Arthur, V. (1995) Written patient information: a review of the literature. *J. Adv. Nurs.* **21**: 1081–1086.

Coulter, A. (1998) Editorial: evidence based patient information. *Br. Med. J.* **317**: 225–226.

Coulter, A., Entwhistle, V. and Gilbert, D. (1998) *Informing Patients*. King's Fund, London.

Gallagher, S. and Zeind, S.M. (1998) Bridging patient education and care. *Am. J. Nurs.* **98**: 16AAA–16DDD.

Goldsborough, R. (1999) Information on the net often needs checking. *RN* **62**: 22–24.

Pennels, C. (2001) Obtaining consent: the use of a consent form. *Prof. Nurse* **16**: 1433–1434.

19 Teaching in Gastroenterology

Harry Dalton, David Levine and Hyder Hussaini

Introduction

The term doctor is derived from the Latin word *docere* – 'to teach'. Doctor is defined by the New Shorter Oxford English Dictionary as 'a person skilled in, and therefore entitled to teach or speak authoritatively on, any branch of knowledge'.

The role of the doctor as an educator goes back to Hippocrates. Doctors taking the Hippocratic oath vowed to teach medicine to the children of the doctors who had taught them. Teaching improves with understanding of educational principles, which we have applied to teaching in gastroenterology.

Teaching endoscopy

The optimum method of teaching endoscopy or assessing trainees' endoscopic skills is not known. In the UK, the BSG recommends that trainees should perform 300 upper GI endoscopies before being allowed to endoscope independently. Whilst this number of procedures may be appropriate for some trainees, others may acquire the appropriate skills before completing 300 procedures, whilst some may take much longer. In addition, there is little emphasis on the actual tuition or assessment that occurs during the '300' procedures. In the era of clinical governance, what is required is a structured method of teaching and a validated means of measuring a trainee's endoscopic skills. Trainees should not be allowed to practice independently until they have passed an assessment of competence using clearly defined, measurable criteria.

There are considerable data from the educational literature regarding the teaching of practical skills. Endoscopy is a practical skill *par excellence* for the gastroenterologist. We decided to apply the educational principles of teaching practical skills to the field of endoscopy. What follows is a description of our current practice, which has been developed over the last few years.

General principles for endoscopy training

Endoscopy is a practical skill that we teach using the four-stage procedure described by Peyton (1998) shown in *Box 19.1*.

This technique can then be applied to any endoscopic procedure, although the procedure may need to be broken down into small 'skill sections' when teaching endoscopy.

The environment for teaching needs to be carefully considered. Adult learners are best taught when not only motivated but also relaxed and free of anxiety. Thus, the training lists should be shorter than nontraining lists. The atmosphere within each training list should be unhurried, with endoscopy assistants who are familiar in the support of the needs of the trainee.

Finally, the attitude of the trainer is key to the success of the training session. The trainer should be a confident, competent endoscopist. However, it is the ability of the trainer to explain endoscopic technique rather than expert technical ability that is important – conscious competence as opposed to unconscious competence.

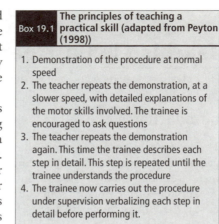

Box 19.1 **The principles of teaching a practical skill (adapted from Peyton (1998))**

1. Demonstration of the procedure at normal speed
2. The teacher repeats the demonstration, at a slower speed, with detailed explanations of the motor skills involved. The trainee is encouraged to ask questions
3. The teacher repeats the demonstration again. This time the trainee describes each step in detail. This step is repeated until the trainee understands the procedure
4. The trainee now carries out the procedure under supervision verbalizing each step in detail before performing it.

The trainer should behave in a manner that avoids fear of failure or humiliation of the trainee, with immediate praise for good technique and positive advice when errors occur. An explanation of procedural technique should be supported by a rationale for the explanation. When a trainee cannot progress during a procedure, the trainer should give the trainee a series of options on how to rectify the problem rather than suggesting a single course of action. All these factors help in the over-riding principle for the trainer – avoid taking the endoscope from the trainee unless there is an absolute need to do so.

The skills that are needed for a trainer in endoscopic procedures highlight the fact that not all competent endoscopists need be involved in training – teaching ability, training and motivation are the key factors for a good teacher of endoscopy. Furthermore, the numbers of trainees that can be trained within an endoscopy unit are limited because the balance of 'service' and 'teaching' lists affects the number of patients undergoing endoscopy. However, teaching endoscopy should be regarded as a core element of the endoscopy 'service'. We therefore limit the number of trainees taught within the unit and have also designated endoscopy trainers, who have both the educational skills and motivation together with endoscopic competence to teach.

Teaching upper gastrointestinal endoscopy

The four phases of teaching upper gastrointestinal endoscopy

To apply the Peyton skill principles to such a complex task as upper GI endoscopy can be difficult. We therefore broke down the procedure into various skill 'sections' and applied the above four-stage procedure to each section. The easiest skill sections are taught first and the hardest (intubation of the esophagus) is taught last. The 13 ground-rules for teaching upper GI endoscopy are:

1. Learners need to be familiar with the endoscope controls
2. Learners need to be relaxed, so do not overbook the list
3. Teach the procedure in skill sections, starting with the easiest first
4. Teach the hardest skill (intubation) last
5. The best place to learn scope control is in the stomach
6. Verbalize intended and completed maneuvers by teacher and learner
7. Give short, precise instructions to the learner
8. Tell your learner to keep off the little wheel as much as possible
9. Say 'well done' to your learner when completing a new maneuver for the first time
10. Do not allow the learner to attempt a complete endoscopy until all the skill sections have been successfully completed
11. The teaching of generic endoscopy skills is an ongoing process
12. The learner must first be able to recognize normality
13. When teaching, **keep your hands off the scope.**

These rules are given to the learner at the beginning of their training. The learner is then taught in four phases.

Phase 1: basic scope control

The trainer shows the trainee the endoscope, how it works and the function of all the controls. We insist that our learners spend a morning cleaning the endoscopes with our endoscopy technician. This helps the learner become familiar with handling the equipment and also gives a basic understanding of infection control. After this, the learner is asked to attend the endoscopy unit for 10 min each day for up to 2 weeks. The purpose of this is to get the learner used to handling the endoscope and to become familiar with the controls in a safe environment away from the patient.

Once the learner has become familiar with handling the endoscope, the teacher demonstrates a full upper GI endoscopy in real time. The teacher then demonstrates the procedure again, but this time gives a full explanation of the maneuvers required to complete each of the five skill sections (J maneuver, withdrawal, duodenal intubation, D2 intubation and gastric biopsy). The teacher demonstrates the procedure again, but this time the learner has to tell the teacher in detail what maneuvers to make in order successfully to complete each skill section. This step is repeated until the learner can accurately verbalize the motor skills and underlying rationale required for each skill section. Finally, the teacher intubates the stomach and the learner takes the scope and performs each skill section verbalizing the intended maneuver before attempting it.

A written record is kept of the learner's progress with regard to their ability to verbalize each skill section followed by the number of successful attempts at each skill (see *Table 19.1*). In our experience phase 1 takes on average 10–20 hands-on procedures to complete.

Table 19.1. Teaching upper gastrointestinal endoscopy: phase 1 evaluation – basic scope control

Skill	Movements	Student able to verbalize	Student able to do (completed/attempted)
J maneuver	Pylorus mid screen Big wheel down Withdraw Right/left torque		
Withdrawal	Blow Do it slow and look Keep off lesser curve with left torque or little wheel down Aspirate excess air before removing scope		
Duodenal intubation	Pylorus mid screen Slowly advance If you lose the view keep still and wait		
D2 intubation	Push 90° clockwise torque Big wheel down		
Gastric biopsy (random)	Open Push Pull Biopsy forcep positioned close to scope tip		
General	Clean lens frequently		

Phase 2: sequential skill sections

The teacher intubates the esophagus. The learner now takes over and passes the endoscope from esophagus to pylorus, and completes the previously learned skills in an increasingly sequential fashion. As the learner is now acquiring better scope control, targeted gastric biopsies are taught at this stage. As in phase 1, before each maneuver, the learner is asked to verbalize any intended adjustment to the endoscope controls and a written record is kept of the learner's progress (*Table 19.2*). Phase 2 takes up to 20 hands-on procedures to learn.

Phase 3: esophageal intubation

The learner now starts to intubate the esophagus, after demonstration by trainer, and verbalization of the trainee's actions for esophageal intubation. Esophageal biopsy is taught at this stage (*Table 19.3*). This stage is the most variable in term of the number of procedures it requires to gain competence. It can take over 50 procedures, but is often much quicker.

Phase 4: full gastroscopy

The learner now performs full upper GI endoscopy. The trainer observes with minimal interference. The learner by now will be able to recognize normality and

Table 19.2. Teaching upper gastrointestinal endoscopy: phase 2 evaluation – sequential skill sections

Skill	Movements	Student able to verbalize	Student able to do (completed/attempted)
J maneuver	Pylorus mid screen Big wheel down Withdraw Right/left torque		
Withdrawal	Blow Do it slow and look Keep off lesser curve with left torque or little wheel down		
Duodenal intubation	Pylorus mid screen Slowly advance If you lose the view keep still and wait		
D2 intubation	Push 90° clockwise torque Big wheel down		
Gastric biopsy (random)	Push Open Pull Biopsy forcep positioned close to scope tip		
Esophagus to pylorus	Push Blow Left torque, then right torque		
Lesion biopsy	Identify abnormal Good tip control Push, open, pull Biopsy forcep positioned close to scope tip		

should be exposed to a varied range of abnormalities as possible. This is achievable if a little thought is given to patient selection for the teaching list.

Teaching colonoscopy

The aim is for trainees to be able to perform total colonoscopy in at least 90% of patients with complete examination of the colonic mucosa in patients who have conscious sedation and for the procedure to be completed in a manner that is safe and comfortable for the patient. The teaching of colonoscopy involves the same general principle outlined previously. The specific nature of colonoscopy training is shown in *Box 19.2*.

There are many variations in technique that will enable the trainee to perform effective and safe colonoscopy. The problem with many techniques is that they are complex and sometimes require tacit knowledge by the operator to be performed successfully. Recently, a joint working party, consisting of expert

Table 19.3. Teaching upper gastrointestinal endoscopy: phase 3 – esophageal intubation

Skill	Movements	Student able to verbalize	Student able to do (completed/attempted)
J maneuver	Pylorus mid screen Big wheel down Withdraw Right/left torque		
Withdrawal	Blow Do it slow and look Keep off lesser curve with left torque or little wheel down		
Duodenal intubation	Pylorus mid screen Slowly advance If you lose the view keep still and wait		
D2 intubation	Push 90° clockwise torque Big wheel down		
Gastric biopsy (random)	Push Open Pull Biopsy forcep positioned close to scope tip		
Esophagus to pylorus	Push Blow Left torque, then right torque		
Lesion biopsy	Identify abnormal Good tip control Push, open, pull Biopsy forcep positioned close to scope tip		
Intubate	Keep in midline Glide over tongue Steady both wheels with left thumb with big wheel down Aim below chords Swallow then gentle push Squirt (+/– blow) then gentle push		
Esophageal biopsy	Spiked forceps Hard down/up on wheel Push, open, pull		

colonoscopists devised a simple algorithm for performing colonoscopy. This is the chosen technique for the accredited regional 'hands-on colonoscopy' courses, organized by the Royal College of Surgeons. These courses follow a set technique protocol with one-to-one 'hands-on' training as opposed to demonstration colonoscopy for trainees. The courses also detail the background knowledge and therapeutic techniques required for colonoscopy. The teaching algorithm has been described recently by Teague *et al.* (2002) and is suggested as further reading in the bibliography. The combination of local teaching and specialized courses according to a national teaching program is probably the way forward for colonoscopy training.

Prior to teaching, trainer and trainee discuss scope handling, verbalization of maneuvers and terminology, and when the trainer may take over during the procedure. As with gastroscopy, the trainer should in general keep hands off the colonoscope during training sessions, although since some problems in colonoscopic advancement are recognized by tactile contact with the scope, this is not always possible. Training lists consist of three to four colonoscopic procedures. The basic skills that we teach in our unit are outlined below.

Box 19.2	Colposcopy training

- Designated colonoscopy teacher and short (3–4 procedures) lists
- Student to be familiar with scope manipulation and verbalization of motor skills
- Techniques to teach
- Sufficient air insufflation
  - Torque steering
  - Loop reduction
  - Suction steering
  - Prevention of loop formation
  - Terminal ileal intubation
  - Scope withdrawal
- Problem recognition and solving
- Feedback
  - During procedure
  - Postcolonoscopy 'debriefing'

Scope handling

The trainees are once again shown the techniques for holding the scope and the nature of the controls. In general, tip angulation is suggested using the up/down control with minimal use of the lateral controls (left/right). Particular emphasis is given to the relationship between angulation of the scope tip and clockwise/counter-clockwise torque. This is important for the techniques of torque steering and loop reduction.

Verbalization of colonoscopy

The trainees are taught to describe verbally what they see on the colonoscopy monitor and their subsequent action. Trainees are taught techniques to identify the lumen, to describe the luminal position in specific relationship to a clock face (e.g. the lumen is at 5 o'clock) and to state their next maneuver with the endoscope controls. In general, this may include tip angulation, torque, suction positional change of the patient and the use of hand pressure to prevent loop re-forming.

Technique

We teach trainees the technique of torque steering in the left colon as this minimizes the formation of loops, although we acknowledge that in some patients (e.g. severe diverticular disease) this may not be possible and steering by tip deflection is needed. In the more proximal colon, a combination of tip angulation with the up/down and lateral controls, suction steering and positional change is used. There is emphasis on appropriate colonic insufflation (but enough to view the lumen), lens washing, maintenance of luminal views and scope position outside the patient (including transference of loop to the umbilicus from the shaft of the scope). Loop recognition is key, with patient discomfort, loss of 1:1 scope advancement, paradoxical movement and general 'tightening' of tip control being suggestive features. Specific techniques such as terminal ileal intubation, prevention of loop re-formation and effective scope withdrawal with appropriate torque need particular instruction.

Problem solving

Problem solving is key to progression during colonoscopy. Thus, the trainee is encouraged to consider different options when a problem is encountered, rather than being told what to do or having the problem overcome by the trainer. For example, when a problem such as loop formation is encountered, the trainee needs to first recognize the problem, then consider the following options: (a) continuation provided there is no excess patient discomfort, (b) clockwise torque and pull back, (c) counter-clockwise torque and pull back or (d) change of patient position into the supine or right lateral position. Thus problem solving during colonoscopy training helps develop confidence and competence in the trainee.

Feedback

Debriefing following each colonoscopy by the trainer gives the trainee the opportunity to express 'what went well' and 'what could be improved' in discussion with the trainer. This reinforces the general principle of praise during the procedure with positive comments on how problems encountered by the trainee can be rectified.

Generic skills in endoscopy

There are a number of skills that the learner will require before becoming competent at any endoscopic technique.

- Appropriateness of the endoscopy
- Likely findings
- Process of informed consent (see Chapter 18)
- Local anesthetic/conscious sedation techniques
- Normal endoscopic appearances
- Communication
  - with the patient
  - writing report (Endoscribe)
- Arrange appropriate treatment and/or follow-up

These skills are taught throughout training, although, in our experience, it is best to concentrate on these aspects of endoscopy once the motor skills for endoscopy have been developed. The reason for this is that initially most learners find mastering the necessary motor skills quite a challenge and trying to teach complex concepts not immediately related to the motor skills required to perform the endoscopy is an unnecessary distraction.

Having used this technique for a while, it is our observation that our trainees seem to enjoy their endoscopy more and become confident more quickly.

Assessment

General principles of assessment

Unlike appraisal, this involves direct comparison of knowledge, skill or behavior with some form of external standard. The comparison may be against one or more of the following:

(a) The measured or perceived level of attainment of the practitioner's peers. (norm-referenced).
(b) An objective criterion that is agreed to a minimum acceptable level. (criterion-referenced).
(c) The personal opinion or judgment of the assessor(s).

(*Note: a, b and c are not always mutually exclusive*).

For any type of assessment, there are two important requirements:

(a) Validity

That is, we are assessing what we claim to assess. One example would be cecal intubation rate in colonoscopy. This is simply and literally a measure of the ability to get to the cecum. Whilst it is a prerequisite for an examination of all the colonic mucosa, it does not in itself tell us anything about the completeness, accuracy or safety of the examination and should not be used as a surrogate for these aspects.

(b) Reliability

That is, the assessment should give similar results if done on another day by another assessor (assuming the practitioner being assessed had not materially improved or deteriorated). This is particularly relevant when assessment contains a significant element of the assessor's personal opinion or judgment. The reliability of this, very common, type of assessment is improved by the use of several assessments done at different times by different people independently. This is important when the result of assessment has long-term consequences.

Although we commonly assume that assessment is simply done as a pass/fail test to tell whether someone is 'good enough', there are other important reasons for assessing. Firstly it may tell us about the adequacy or otherwise of a training program. We should not assume that everyone has been properly taught what is being assessed. Secondly, the results of assessments should be used to help the practitioner improve. This requires skilful feedback of assessment results. One simple but effective technique is first to discuss specifically what was done well and then to discuss what specifically needs to be improved. The emphasis on 'improvement' is considerably more motivating than talking about 'weakness' or what was 'bad'. The results of assessments are therefore a vital component of appraisal.

Whilst we would like to think that an assessment will predict future success, this is often unrealistic. Experience shows that, like the stock market, past performance can be a poor guide to future returns. To some extent, this can be improved by making assessment, like appraisal, a long intudinal process rather than a snapshot. We must, however, recognize the difference between competence and performance. Competence is about someone's capabilities under conditions that are relatively controlled and favorable, whilst performance day to day has to contend with the multitude of personal and extraneous factors that can affect outcomes for even the most competent of individuals.

Finally, even when assessments have been designed to include all the above features they have to be affordable and feasible as well as acceptable to those involved.

Assessment in gastrointestinal endoscopy

Despite the huge numbers of procedures being performed, and the many endoscopists learning and performing the procedures, there is still no generally accepted method of assessing endoscopic skills. To some extent, this reflects a lack of agreed standards. Because of this, it is likely that individual units and trainers will, for the foreseeable future need to design their own methods and be prepared to modify them in the light of experience and new knowledge. For those intending to carry out assessments for the first time, there are techniques and approaches that may make the process more effective and rewarding:

General points

- Be aware of the type(s) of assessment you are using and recognize that even when you are ostensibly using 'norm-' or 'criterion-referenced' assessment there is often still a large element of personal opinion or judgment. This is not necessarily a bad thing but may need to be made more explicit and reproducible. Perhaps the most rigorous assessment is for you to decide whether we would want that person performing an endoscopy on you.
- Remind yourself regularly how to give feedback.
- Assess specifically what has been taught. This also emphasizes the need, often forgotten, to make it known at the start of a training program, that the learner will be assessed on what is taught.
- Make frequent and unthreatening short assessments part of day-to-day teaching and learning. Direct these formative assessments at specific sections of the procedure before assessing the full procedure. This will make any 'final' or summative assessment easier and avoid surprises.
- Try to separate process and outcome assessments:

(a) Your assessments of knowledge, skill and attitude under observation are tests of competence. They can be supplemented by feedback from patients, nurses and other staff but this feedback should still be in the form described above. Beware of feedback that reflects personal likes and dislikes rather than modifiable observed behavior.

(b) Outcome assessments could include accuracy, missed lesions and complications. These are all suitable for audit but the lack of good information systems can hamper this work.

- Make clear in advance what is to be assessed. At least for summative assessments try to use a proforma. You need to be clear before you start what you are assessing and to keep to a plan.
- Demonstrate that you, as a trainer, are willing to undergo direct assessment of your endoscopic skill as well as auditing your outcomes. Many older consultants are largely self-taught and few undergo rigorous peer review. It can be a liberating experience but the rules on feedback are the same as for trainees!

Cusum analysis

This is a technique for monitoring performance over time. It is an established method of quality control in laboratories and has more recently been evaluated in clinical practice, particularly to assess whether defined standards of skill are being reached. The method involves calculating a *cu*mulative *sum* of scores for success or failure in a procedure. According to the standard involved a positive score is assigned to a failure and a negative score to a success or vice versa (depending on which direction you want the curve to take). In colonoscopy, it is proving useful in assessing whether the endoscopist is reaching and maintaining the required 90% standard for examination to the cecum (JAG (2001)). In this case, each failure is assigned +0.9 and each success −0.1. Achieving a steady-state horizontal line indicates that the standard is being maintained (see *Figure 19.1*). The technique is easily put into an Excel program on a personal disk for each endoscopist who simply enters each procedure as a success or failure. The resulting graph can be updated as needed, and provides much better evidence of proficiency than simply a stated success rate without reference to time or number of procedures. The maintenance of a personal cusum chart also provides motivating feedback and prompt indication of need for more training.

Teaching in clinic

Postgraduates

In an ideal world, the four-phase model (see *Box 19.3*) should be used to guide the postgraduate education of junior staff in clinic. In the real world of a bustling gastroenterology outpatient clinic, this is, however, rarely (if ever) possible. There are alternatives to this labor-intensive process, which are relatively straightforward to arrange and do not significantly interfere with the throughput of patients.

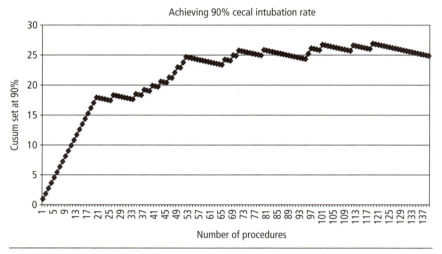

Figure 19.1. A cusum chart

This is a typical cusum analysis of a learner being trained in colonoscopy. The first part of the curve (procedures 1–20) has a steep slope and represents repeated failure to intubate the cecum. Following additional, structured intensive training, the curve flattens out as the learner more consistently reaches the cecum. After 70 procedures this trainee consistently reaches the cecum in 90% of cases (the curve is flat). Thanks to Dr Sue Turner for agreeing to the use of her cusum chart.

Hot review

At the end of the clinic, the trainer and learner get together with all the case notes of the patients seen by the learner. The trainer asks the learner to give a 40-second thumbnail sketch of the case, the decisions made and the clinical reasoning behind these decisions. Most of the cases will have been straightforward, but there will be one or two cases that will bring up issues worthy of further discussion. These issues can be discussed at the time, if time permits. However, it may be better to ask the trainee to reflect on the issues involved and do some reading around the subject. Hot review when used in this way is, therefore, mainly a method of helping the learner identify their learning needs.

| Box 19.3 | **A model for outpatient teaching** |

The following four-phase model can guide education in the outpatient setting:

1. A clinician (preferably the learner's supervisor) demonstrates some clinical practice, which the trainee observes and then discusses with the clinician
2. The learner reflects on these observations and discussions, and 'captures the learning' through reading and writing
3. The learner practices while being supervised by the clinician who gives constructive feedback on the trainee's performance
4. The learner performs unsupervised, though with continuing support, and has opportunities to discuss his or her performance with the supervisor

Adapted from Peyton (1998).

Video consultations

Videotaping outpatient consultations can be a useful technique for developing complex interpersonal skills such as consultation, communication skills and the breaking of bad news. This is clearly much more economical in terms of time than sitting in clinic with the learner and observing directly. It also allows the learner a unique insight as to how they come across to the patient. Another advantage is that the learner can take the video away and reflect on the contents at home. Being videotaped doing a consultation is a soul-baring experience, and when you see yourself on video for the first time it can be quite challenging.

Videotaping has been extensively used in general practice for many years but is now being increasingly used in secondary care. It is really only useful for developing complex interpersonal skills. Other skills such as subject knowledge and clinical decision-making are clearly best taught using different techniques. The logistics of setting up the camera can be problematic, but the rewards seem worth it. Some patients and doctors find the presence of cameras rather intimidating, and it is essential to obtain proper written consent from the patient before *and after* the consultation. An example of the consent form we use is shown in *Figure 19.2*.

Undergraduates

The traditional model for undergraduate teaching in the outpatient clinic is that the students sit in with the consultant and observe the proceedings. This passive role has only limited educational value, as it is well established that adult learners learn best when they are actively engaged. This is rarely the case when the above model is employed. There are, however, several methods of actively engaging students in outpatients.

With final-year students, we find it useful to allow the student to see one or two new patients. Consent is first obtained and it is explained in detail that the patient will first see the student and then the consultant and student together. The student then goes off to see the patient in a separate consulting room with instructions to perform a history and examination. To focus the student we usually set a time limit of 40 min. After this time, the student reports back to the consultant and briefly presents the history and examination findings. The consultant then goes with the student to see the patient and does a normal consultation with the student observing. Once the patient has left, there follows a 5-min discussion with the student about the case. Most students find this immensely valuable and it is relatively economical in consultant time, adding no more than 20 min to the average clinic.

With more junior clinical students, the above technique is inappropriate. One model that can be used is as follows. If there are five doctors doing an outpatient clinic each week, one of the five doctors takes it in turn to teach and do nothing else for that clinic. The other four colleagues doing the clinic identify patients who are suitable and willing to be taught on. The patient is then sent through to the teaching area to meet the students and the teacher. There then follows a bedside clinical teaching session. This is repeated several times during the clinic,

VIDEO
RECORDING OF CONSULTATIONS
PATIENT INFORMATION

We are asking you for your consent to video your consultation.

1. The recording is to help the doctor learn more about how he/she consults and communicates with patients in order to improve patient care.

2. This tape may be seen by health professionals working in the same team.

3. The tape will be kept securely and wiped clean within one year.

4. No embarrassing or intimate examinations will be recorded.

5. You have the opportunity to change your mind after your consultation.

6. Your consultation will be the same as it would have been without the recording.

7. Parents of children under 16 or carer's of patients with learning difficulties or with difficulty in understanding the implications of being recorded must give their consent.

It is natural to have concerns about being filmed or observed, especially during a private meeting with a doctor and we fully understand if you prefer not to be recorded.

It is important to realise that the doctor will not mind either way and that your treatment or subsequent consultations will not be influenced in any way by what you decide.

Thank you for your help and co-operation.

I agree to the Royal Cornwall Hospitals Trust taking a video of me during a teaching session for student doctors while in the Trust's care. I understand the video will be used in support of teaching work on behalf of the Trust and agree the Trust will have sole discretion in the use of the video.

I understand that at the end of this video if I so wish I may withdraw my permission *

Signed_____ Date_____

Print_____ CR No:_____

*I withdraw my permission for this video: Signed_____

                                            Date_____

Figure 19.2. Video for teaching agreement

and quite a number of patients with varying physical signs can be seen and taught on in a single clinical session. Up to six students can be taught at a time. This is a very effective way of teaching but is labor-intensive. In the above scenario, the throughput of the clinic will go down by 20% as a direct result of the teaching. This is clearly only sustainable when such teaching is properly funded by the parent university.

Teaching on the ward round

Postgraduates

There has been an inexorable year-on-year increase in the volume of general medical inpatient work, largely as a result of a sustained increase in the number of emergency medical admissions. This makes general physicians busy people, and gastroenterologists are no exception. It is not uncommon for a business ward round to include over 30 patients on several different wards and take up to 3 h to complete. For the gastroenterologist to fulfill his/her teaching role in this situation can be problematic due to the volume of work and lack of time. It is common to hear the mantra 'business rounds are for business, not for teaching'. However, recent work at our institution concerning how junior doctors learn has challenged this idea.

Provisional data from a study looking at the ward round as a teaching vehicle has produced interesting results. The ward round is a poor way of transmitting knowledge to junior staff, but it is an excellent way of teaching professionalization, making the change from student to doctor. In other words, the ward round can be regarded as a rite of passage in the learner's professional development. This includes areas such as communication skills, clinical decision-making and professional attitudes. In some ways, whatever the format of the business round, it will have a major educational component in the above terms.

Understanding the educational role of the business round is important for two reasons. Firstly, it is a poor way of transmitting knowledge, which should be learnt and taught using different techniques. Secondly, it is likely that generating the correct atmosphere on the business round is key to maximizing its educational effectiveness. The best way of doing this remains to be determined.

Undergraduates

In our opinion, business rounds are inappropriate for most medical students. The exception to this is final-year students who are learning medicine in the apprenticeship style. Such students may get significant educational value from a business round, if they are treated as the junior member of the team and actively engaged in the process. It needs to be remembered, however, that the educational value to the student will mainly be in the area of the development of professional attitudes rather than knowledge (see above).

Clinical skills and knowledge are best taught to undergraduates by a dedicated teaching round. We have given the format of this teaching round considerable thought over the last few years. Our current practice, whose major aim is to teach clinical examination skills of the GI system, is described in detail below:

- Four patients (inpatients on the gastroenterology ward) are chosen, consented and briefed.
- Sixteen students arrive and are briefed and split up into four groups of four students each.

- The aims of the session are clarified verbally.
- Each group is taught by a member of the gastroenterology team (consultants or specialist/research registrars). This involves each group seeing each patient in turn in a 'round robin' fashion.
- One student is chosen to perform a physical examination of the GI tract. The other three students are asked to actively observe.
- When the student has finished the physical examination feedback is given using a nonthreatening 'Pendleton'-style approach from:
  - The patient
  - The other students
  - The teacher

The student is then asked to describe his/her findings and to discuss aspects of the case. The teacher often follows this by a 2-min microteaching session on the topic. The advantages of this approach are:

- All learners take an active role, even if they physically do not get 'hands-on'.
- Students reflect on their own practice by giving feedback to others.
- Patients take an active role in the teaching process by giving feedback to the students. This stops them from being a 'commodity' and personalizes the process for the student.
- Each student gets 'hands-on' at least once.
- The session is taught by a team. This has been helpful in terms of team building and staff educational development, as the session is videotaped every 6 months and we discuss the process as a team.
- Because we teach as a team, the teaching session is sustainable. If a member of staff is absent someone else fills in, or the students are redistributed to the number of teachers available. This means that the teaching session is rarely, if ever, canceled.

Conclusions

Gastroenterologists are involved in teaching in many ways. It is important for the teacher to appreciate the principles of adult education as applied to gastro-enterology. This will allow the learner to gain maximum benefit from the considerable effort that has been invested in the educational process.

There are many demands on a gastroenterologist's time. To address all the above educational issues correctly not only takes a lot of thought, but also involves considerable time. We believe that the only way this can be achieved is by having properly protected and funded fixed educational sessions in the consultant gastroenterologist's work plan. General practice have realized for years that educational time needs to be properly protected and funded. This is a lesson that secondary care needs to learn.

Further reading

Peyton, J.W.R. (1998) *Teaching and Learning in Medical Practice.* Manticore Europe Limited, Rickmansworth, UK.

Teague, R.H., Soehendra, N., Carr-Locke, D., Segal, E., Sakai, Y., Chao, W. and Nagy, G. (2002) Setting standards in colonoscopic teaching and training. *J. Gastroenterol. Hepatol.*, in press.

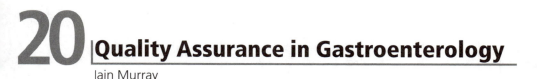

Quality Assurance in Gastroenterology

Iain Murray

Introduction

In recent years, quality of care in the health service has come under increasing public scrutiny. It is high on both political and public agendas because of several high profile cases. As a result, the government, through the Department of Health, the General Medical Council (GMC) and the Royal Colleges have all produced initiatives to increase transparency in the process and quality of healthcare.

To insure quality, an acceptable standard of care has to be agreed. Regular auditing of performance, by both individuals and groups, provides assurance that these standards are being met. Standards need to be clinically relevant and achievable. Their monitoring should be followed by a continuous cycle of improvements and review.

Setting the standards

Endoscopy

The Joint Advisory Group on Gastrointestinal Endoscopy (JAG) has produced guidelines for the training, appraisal and assessment of trainees. These state the minimum requirements for a unit to be accredited for training any endoscopist (specialist registrar, clinical assistant or nurse endoscopist). JAG represents all UK Royal Colleges of Physicians and Surgeons as well as the Royal Colleges of Radiologists and General Practitioners. Although these are standards for training accreditation, they also provide written standards of competence to be accepted before independently performing procedures (see *Table 20.1*). These standards are uniform for all endoscopy practitioners including medical, surgical and nurse endoscopists and radiologists performing endoscopy.

Outpatients

Audit of quality of healthcare provision is especially difficult in outpatients. Correspondingly, there are few written guidelines regarding standards.

The Patients' Charter does state that new patients graded urgent should be seen within 2 weeks, those graded soon within 4 weeks and within 13 weeks for routine. Patients should be seen within 30 min of their appointment time or given a reasonable explanation.

Table 20.1. Acceptable standards for independent endoscopic practitioners based on JAG guidelines (2001)

Generic standards

- Understanding of indications and contra-indications for each type of endoscopic procedure
- Knowledge and skills in conscious sedation and management of sedation-related complications and their avoidance
- Knowledge of causes, recognition and management of endoscopy-related complications and their avoidance
- Principles and practice of informed consent
- Communicating endoscopic findings to patients and carers, including giving 'bad news'
- Knowledge of current surveillance protocols

Esophagogastroduodenoscopy	Colonoscopy	ERCP
• High success rate in intubating patients with minimal trauma and discomfort	• Cecal utubation rates exceeding 90% in patients without colonic strictures or fecal contamination	• Selectively cannulate required duct in 90% of cases and provide biliary drainage
• High success rate in intubating pylorus	• Terminal ileal intubation rate exceeding 50% in those patients in whom it is indicated	• Interpret radiological findings and assess significance of these in context of patient's illness
• Ability to visualize endoscopic blind spots	• Ability to perform hot biopsy, polypectomy and techniques to control bleeding	• Perform endoscopic sphincterotomy
• Inject bleeding lesions, band varices and use thermal methods to stop bleeding	• Balloon dilatation of strictures and treatment of angiodysplastic lesions	
• Dilate esophageal strictures	• Dye spraying, tattooing, endoscopic mucosal resection, tumor debulking and stenting (not all practitioners need these skills)	
• Remove foreign objects		
• Insert percutaneous endoscopic gastrostomy tubes and knowledge of associated ethical issues		
• Palliate esophagogastric malignancy (stents, thermal ablative techniques and dilatation)		
• Polypectomy (including knowledge of endoscopic mucosal resection)		
• Knowledge of complications of therapeutic techniques		

More recently, the Government has guaranteed that any patient suspected of having cancer would be seen by a specialist within 2 weeks of the intention to refer. This has led to many local initiatives to speed up referrals. These include asking Primary Care Groups to fax requests to dedicated machines, establishing generic lists to enable patients to be seen within the specified time and nurse specialists running these generic clinic lists. Local service provision will dictate whether patients are seen for a definitive investigation or for outpatient review as their first appointment. Ideally, a one-stop clinic will permit patients to be assessed, investigated and given reassurance. Their further management can be planned and discussed. Provision of these new rapid access services without detriment to those referred by other mechanisms is an impossible task without additional funding.

Emphasis is placed on making a patient-centered NHS: one of the cornerstones of the work of the Commission for Health Improvement (CHI). It is likely that patient questionnaires on their satisfaction with their outpatient clinic review will become mandatory.

The Royal Colleges encourage senior house officers to see both new and returning patients in clinics. However, there must be adequate supervision preferably by a consultant or at least a specialist registrar. Senior house officers can only see patients alone if the consultant has reviewed the case notes beforehand. Clinics should include adequate time for the senior house officer to present and discuss patient management. Consultants should see a maximum of eight new patients or 20 follow-up patients per clinic, with doctors in training seeing a maximum of half this number.

Auditing outcomes

Endoscopy

It is comparatively easy to audit immediate outcomes in endoscopy. Suitable subjects should be clinically relevant and measurable. These could include completion rates for colonoscopy (cusum analysis, see Chapter 19, Assessment in gastrointestinal endoscopy) selective cannulation rates for ERCP and achieving biliary drainage. Sedation use (including patients' oxygen saturation during the procedure) and patient perception of discomfort during procedures, explanation and preparedness for procedures and immediate complication rates could all be audited. Such information will become essential in future for an endoscopy unit to be accredited for both training and possibly performing procedures.

Equally important, but more difficult to document, are the late-complication and 30-day mortality rates. It would require increased resources to obtain this information for endoscopic procedures as is done for the National Confidential Enquiry into Peri-operative Deaths (NCEPOD). The incidence of missed diagnoses is equally important, but again has major funding implications.

Outpatients

It is relatively easy to audit new patient referral waiting time for their first appointment, the numbers of new and returning patients seen and to seek service user feedback on the services provided. However, it is more important to audit the quality rather than the quantity of the service and this is more difficult. One method is peer review of case notes to determine if appropriate information was obtained, the extent of examination performed and details of investigations requested. Peer review of outpatient consultations, either by observation during a clinic or by video-recording consultations for later review (both with informed patient consent), would be more meaningful but require greater resources.

Patient feedback on the service provided should be wide-ranging, including information on processes, as well as their views on the quality of their consultation.

Mechanisms of quality assurance

Annual appraisal

All consultants will be appraised annually by their peers within the Trust. Appraisers are appointed by, and fulfill a management function on behalf of, the chief executive. The chief executive should assure him/herself that the appraisers have appropriate skills and training for the task. Before being appraised, the consultant constructs a learning portfolio, and gains a written report from their clinical director. Feedback is also obtained from other members of the clinical teams.

The learning portfolios of experienced consultants should be used to confirm good professional practice, as laid down by the GMC, and demonstrate lifelong learning. The essentials of a learning profile are:

- Personal details, including details of previous posts and membership of societies
- Details of current medical activities, including subspecialist skills and commitments, details of emergency, on-call and out-of-hours responsibilities, outpatient work, other clinical work, teaching and academic work
- Examples of good medical care, including current job plan, information on annual workload/caseload, audit data, evidence of how audit has resulted in changes in practice, results of clinical outcomes, evidence of resource shortfalls which compromise outcomes, in-service educational activity and effect on service delivery, the outcome of investigated formal complaints within the previous 12 months, how complaints have affected practice, outcome of external peer review, issues in relation to employer clinical governance policies, evidence of clinical guideline review and how they affect practice and critical incident reports
- Examples of maintaining good medical practice, including CPD/CME activities and difficulty in attending CPD/CME activities if relevant

- Reflection on working relationships with colleagues including description of work setting and team structure (including formal peer reviews)
- Evidence of good relations with patients and description of handling informed consent (patient surveys, changes in practice after complaint, peer reviews/surveys)
- A summary of teaching and training activities
- Issues regarding probity and health
- Formal management activities, noteworthy achievements and feedback
- Research commitments

The primary purpose of the assessment should be improvement in the individual's (and clinical team's) practice with development actions agreed and acted upon. In a very few cases, it may become apparent that an individual's practice fails to meet an acceptable standard and remedial action, and possibly even censure, becomes necessary; in other words, in most cases assessment should be formative rather than summative.

Revalidation

The GMC has been given the role of overseeing revalidation. All practicing doctors, not in training posts, will be assessed to determine their fitness to practice and their continued registration. The aim is to identify those who are poorly performing, to promote good practice and increase public confidence in doctors. It is promised that the process will be effective, transparent, comprehensive, thorough, proportionate, fair, nondiscriminatory, consistent and verifiable. It will also compare a doctor's actual practice to national standards.

Revalidation is likely to commence in 2004 and will take three stages:

1. A folder of information reviewed regularly (by annual appraisal, see Annual appraisal, above), describing what a doctor does
2. Periodic revalidation by a group of medical and lay people (probably two doctors and one layperson). They will use a summary of these personal portfolios and outcomes of annual appraisals to recommend whether registration with the GMC continue or be reviewed
3. The GMC will either confirm continued registration or perform detailed investigations to determine fitness to practice

The Seven Cornerstones of good medical practice, according to the GMC, are:

- Good professional practice
- Maintaining good medical practice
- Relationship with patients
- Working with colleagues
- Teaching and training
- Health
- Probity

For most doctors, there should be minimal effort involved beyond compiling a yearly personal portfolio for appraisal (above) and completing forms regarding health and probity.

Commission for Health Improvement

The CHI is a statutory independent review body set up by government in 1999 to improve patient care in the NHS in England and Wales. It plans to carry out routine clinical governance review of all NHS organizations every 4 years.

Each review consists of preparation, a week-long visit by CHI auditors, then report. At the preparation stage, information on data, minutes and complaints (mostly already in the public domain) are compiled. The information is reviewed to identify areas of best practice and areas for improvement.

The review will assess 'the patient's experience' looking at their 'journey' through the organization, the outcome of their treatment, their views and opinions and the environment in which they were treated. The clinical teams will also be reviewed and systems and processes examined to determine how they influence patient care. Finally, corporate strategy is examined, particularly risk management, complaints handling, patient involvement, research and clinical effectiveness, clinical audit, information management and human resource management. The outcome of a CHI review will not be incriminatory of individuals but report on good and poor processes, and systems of care.

Adverse events reporting

It is essential in an organization that every member of staff feels able to report, in a nonthreatening environment, any incident which they consider compromises the quality of patient care. The idea is that the NHS is to be 'an organization with a memory'. Adverse events reporting should permit the organization to learn from the event and improve the systems that have caused the event. It should not sanction individuals. Lessons from some adverse events may be disseminated throughout the Trust or even through the NHS as a whole, if similar problems could arise elsewhere. Feedback must be given to the staff reporting the event to ensure that they are aware of changes arising from their report and are encouraged to report on any further adverse events.

Clinical governance meetings

Each NHS Trust is required to 'put and keep in place arrangements for the purpose of monitoring and improving the quality of care which it provides to individuals' [Health Act 1999, Duty of Quality 18(1)].

Gastroenterologists will be expected to take part in clinical governance within the medical directorate, although larger units may wish to have independent clinical governance meetings in view of the unique nature of their posts. Guidelines from appropriate sources (e.g. NICE, BSG, Royal Colleges) should be disseminated, reviewed and implemented. Audit should be planned and reported and areas of 'good practice' implemented throughout the Trust.

As mentioned previously, clinical governance requires enhanced patient/user involvement in Trust activity. This means actively seeking public/service users' views in planning services and in delivery of care as well as actively seeking feedback on service provision. Complaints should be discussed to determine if there have been system failures and to promote improvement in service provision.

Risk management must include a review of clinical practice, reporting and review of deaths, and critical incidents within the unit.

Conclusions

Transparent quality assurance for the medical profession is important today and will become increasingly so. The exact nature by which quality assurance is measured and demonstrated will evolve and may differ from those processes described here. Clear and complete documentation of work performed will be needed. Exact details for each NHS organization should be obtainable from clinical directors with further details from such organizations as the GMC, British Medical Association, BSG and the Royal Colleges.

Useful websites

www.gmc-uk.org
www.bma.org.uk
www.bsg.org.uk
www.rcplondon.ac.uk
www.rcpsglasg.ac.uk
www.rcpe.ac.uk

Further reading

Joint Advisory Group On Gastrointestinal Endoscopy (1999)
Recommendations for training in gastrointestinal endosopy.

21 | Radiology and the Gastroenterology Team

Richard Farrow and Giles Maskell

Introduction

In recent years, the role of imaging has become ever more important in the care of patients with a wide range of GI problems, and gastroenterologists have become accustomed to working closely with colleagues in the radiology department. At its simplest level, this can involve a weekly clinicoradiological meeting, but this can evolve into much closer patterns of working between the two departments to the benefit of patients. Integrated investigation pathways can be developed for patients with conditions such as jaundice, dysphagia and IDA. Such close working links are greatly facilitated if the endoscopy unit is in close proximity to the radiology department and particularly the fluoroscopy facility, where barium studies are performed.

Fluoroscopy (X-ray screening) is mandatory for many therapeutic endoscopy procedures such as ERCP and is extremely helpful for others including esophageal dilatation and stent insertion. This can be achieved either by the use of a dedicated fluoroscopy room within the X-ray department for these procedures or by employing a mobile image intensifier and radiographer. This shared use of facilities and staff also helps to foster team working between the GI unit and X-ray department.

The following sections contain a brief overview of current imaging pathways for a range of common GI problems, but there can be no substitute for face-to-face discussion between the clinician and radiologist over individual cases.

Gastrointestinal bleeding

The investigation of obscure GI bleeding is often a challenge to both radiologist and gastroenterologist, and close collaboration is required if the diagnosis is to be reached with the minimum of invasive tests.

In the acute setting, if the site of blood loss is felt to be in the upper GI tract, then the first investigation is endoscopy to evaluate the esophagus, stomach and duodenum. If this investigation fails to reveal a source for the bleeding, such as ulceration or mucosal tear, then additional radiological studies will be required. Investigations that may help include nuclear medicine studies or mesenteric angiography, but the choice will require close liaison with the radiology department. In patients with continuing GI bleeding, the investigation of choice is a mesenteric angiogram with selective catheterization of the celiac, superior mesenteric and inferior mesenteric vessels. This will detect a bleeding site in about 90% of patients if the rate of blood loss is greater than 0.5 ml min^{-1} (*Figure 21.1*). In more chronic blood loss, nuclear medicine studies with technetium-labeled erythrocytes have an established place in diagnosis. Once a bleeding site has been identified, an angiogram is often required to localize more precisely the bleeding point. Occasionally a tumor blush will reveal the diagnosis, even when no active bleeding is demonstrated. If this fails to detect an abnormality, consideration should be given to evaluating the small bowel with a small bowel enteroclysis.

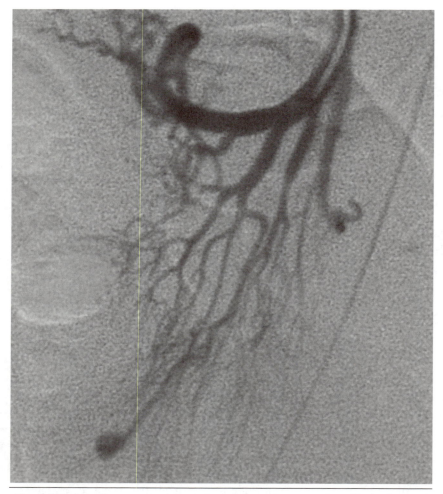

Figure 21.1. Selective superior mesenteric angiogram demonstrating a blush of contrast due to a small bowel arterio-venous malformation.

In patients with acute bleeding from the lower GI tract, colonoscopy can be extremely useful but can be very difficult because the colon is unprepared, and other studies such as angiography or nuclear medicine can be helpful.

In patients with assumed chronic GI blood loss who present with IDA, the whole of the GI tract needs to be examined. Patients should have an upper GI endoscopy to examine the esophagus, stomach and duodenum. These patients should have biopsies of the second part of the duodenum so that a diagnosis of celiac disease can be made or excluded. Even if a lesion is identified at upper GI endoscopy, the colon still requires evaluation. In fit patients, most centers would offer either a colonoscopy or a combined flexible sigmoidoscopy and double contrast barium enema. The choice between these tests depends greatly on local provision. Colonoscopy allows the assessment of finer mucosal detail than a barium enema and can also treat a variety of conditions during the same visit. The barium enema is, however, a statistically safer test, which has a higher chance of adequately examining the whole colon. The use of carbon dioxide as the insufflating gas allows a high-quality barium enema to be performed on the same day as a flexible sigmoidoscopy due to the rapid clearance of gas. This is a significant advantage in that it reduces the number of visits that patients need to make to the hospital. Increasingly a virtual colonoscopy technique using CT is used as an alternative (*Figure 21.2*). In this test, the patient has full bowel preparation and rectal gas followed by abdominal CT in both the prone and supine positions. The colon can then be assessed for mucosal lesions. This test has the advantage of showing a range of extraluminal disease that may be clinically significant. In patients who are very immobile, a CT scan with minimal patient preparation can be used. The patient is given oral contrast to drink the night before the examination in addition to the standard preparation. CT will then demonstrate most significant colonic pathology (*Figure 21.3*) with minimal discomfort for the patient.

In patients with suspected GI bleeding in whom the diagnosis still remains unclear, small bowel enteroclysis is indicated. This will detect small bowel tumors as nodular fold thickening or as a focal stricture (*Figure 21.4*) and will also exclude CD. If this test is also negative, then a pertechnetate scan to look for heterotopic gastric mucosa within a Meckel's diverticulum may occasionally be helpful.

Abdominal pain or mass

In clinical practice, the choice of imaging investigation will vary depending on factors in the history and the examination findings. If the history is suggestive of ureteric colic, for example, a plain abdominal radiograph and intravenous urogram (IVU) would be appropriate. For most patients with upper abdominal pain, however, the first imaging test will be an ultrasound scan. This is about 98% accurate for the diagnosis of gallstones and provides a useful overview of the upper abdominal organs including liver, pancreas, spleen and kidneys. In patients with a negative EGD, ultrasound scan and persistent pain, particularly if pancreatic disease is suspected, CT scan should be the next investigation. This is very sensitive for the detection of pancreatic calcification (*Figure 21.5*), which

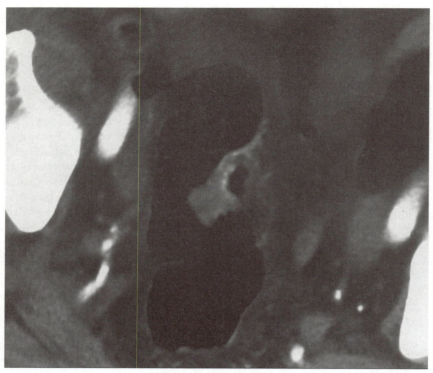

Figure 21.2. Computed tomography with rectal gas demonstrating a pedunculated polyp.

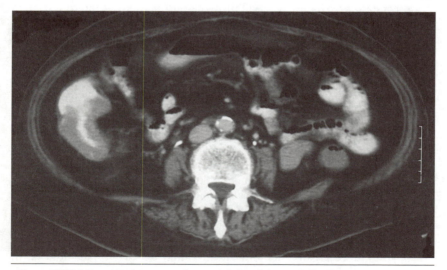

Figure 21.3(a) Computed tomography scan of the abdomen following an oral contrast the previous day. This shows thickening of the wall of the cecum due to a carcinoma.

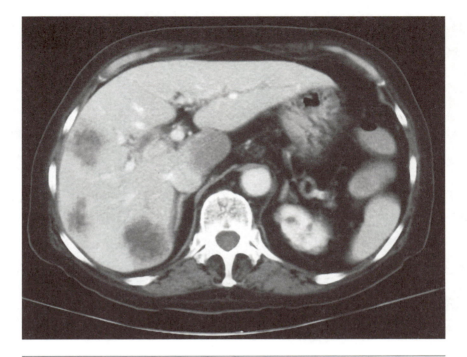

Figure 21.3(b). The same scan demonstrates multiple liver metastases.

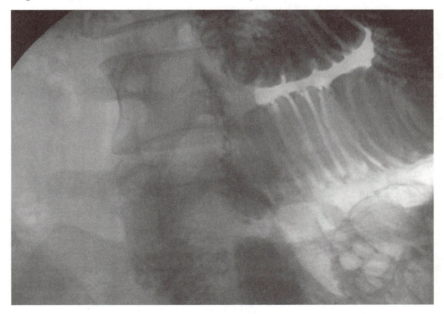

Figure 21.4. Small bowel enema (enteroclysis) demonstrating a jejunal stricture.

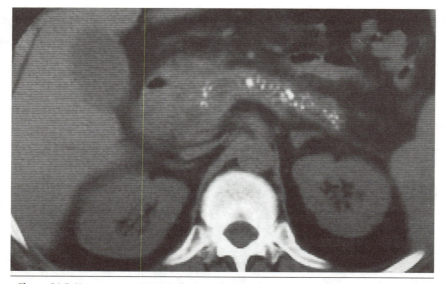

Figure 21.5. Noncontrast computed tomography scan of the abdomen on a patient with abdominal pain demonstrating pancreatic calcification in a patient with chronic pancreatitis.

can be difficult to recognize on ultrasound, and will also identify most tumors of the exocrine pancreas.

For patients with lower abdominal pain, ultrasound is again usually the best initial imaging technique, particularly in the assessment of the female pelvis. Transvaginal ultrasound scanning improves visualization of the pelvic organs in most women and can be carried out without bladder filling. In patients with symptoms suggestive of bowel obstruction, a plain radiograph of the abdomen should be performed. Small bowel obstruction can be assessed further with either CT or barium studies such as enteroclysis. When pain is thought to be of colonic origin, imaging of the large bowel can be performed either with colonoscopy or barium enema.

In patients with acute severe abdominal pain, the 'acute abdomen', the principal decision required for management is whether to proceed to surgery. In the past, this decision was usually made by the surgeon on the basis of history, examination, blood tests and plain films alone. There is now an increasing tendency to employ further imaging in the acute setting to aid this decision. CT scan is highly accurate in the diagnosis (*Figure 21.6*) of a variety of entities including appendicitis, obstruction, diverticulitis and acute bowel ischemia, all of which can present in this way. A negative CT scan may also be used to support a decision to defer surgery and will reduce the number of 'negative laparotomies'.

Abdominal masses can be readily assessed with either ultrasound or CT (*Figure 21.7*). CT is usually more helpful when the mass is arising from or related to bowel and is also more reliable in excluding the presence of a mass when none is present.

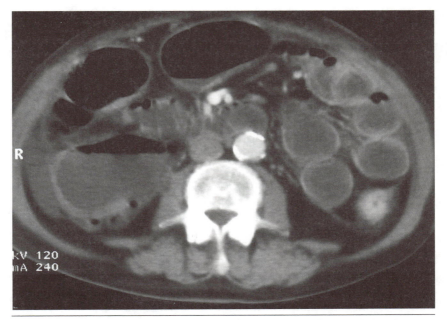

Figure 21.6. Computed tomography scan of the abdomen demonstrating dilated large and small bowel due to an obstructing carcinoma in the left colon.

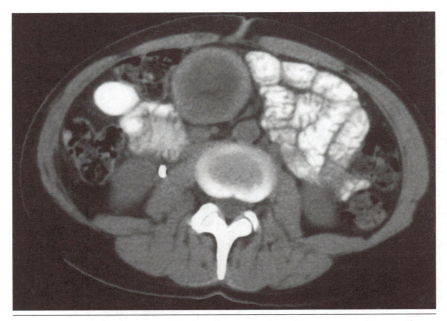

Figure 21.7. Computed tomography scan demonstrating a large mesenteric mass. There is also a right ureteric stent in place.

The jaundiced patient

The first imaging investigation in a jaundiced patient should be an ultrasound examination of the upper abdomen. The scan should be performed in optimal conditions with the patient fasted for at least 6 h to ensure an empty stomach and maximal distention of the gallbladder (see *Box 21.1*). The primary objective of the ultrasound scan is to determine whether the bile ducts are dilated although much other useful information can be obtained and the underlying cause of an obstructive jaundice can often be established with considerable accuracy (*Figure 21.8*). Obstructive jaundice can certainly occur without dilated bile ducts, especially in the early stages of obstruction and in patients with underlying chronic liver disease, but for practical purposes, a normal ultrasound scan should prompt a search for a hepato-

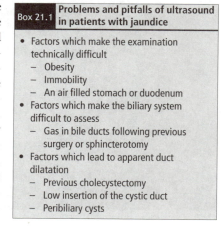

Box 21.1	Problems and pitfalls of ultrasound in patients with jaundice

- Factors which make the examination technically difficult
  - Obesity
  - Immobility
  - An air filled stomach or duodenum
- Factors which make the biliary system difficult to assess
  - Gas in bile ducts following previous surgery or sphincterotomy
- Factors which lead to apparent duct dilatation
  - Previous cholecystectomy
  - Low insertion of the cystic duct
  - Peribiliary cysts

cellular cause for the jaundice. If there is continuing clinical suspicion of an obstructive cause, a repeat scan after 48 h may be worthwhile.

In a jaundiced patient without dilated bile ducts, ultrasound may still provide useful clues to the diagnosis including evidence of portal hypertension, focal liver lesions or other evidence of metastases or splenomegaly.

If dilated bile ducts are demonstrated, it is usually possible to determine whether the level of obstruction is at the porta hepatis or within the common

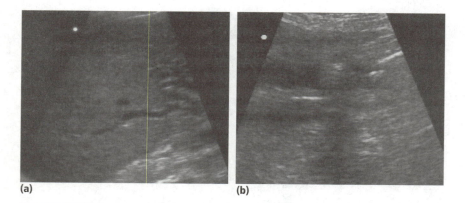

(a) (b)

Figure 21.8. Ultrasound demonstrating dilated intrahepatic bile ducts (a) and a stone in the common bile duct (b). A subsequent endoscopic cholangiogram confirms the findings (c).

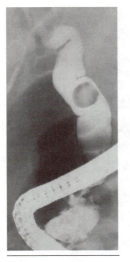

Figure 21.8 (c).

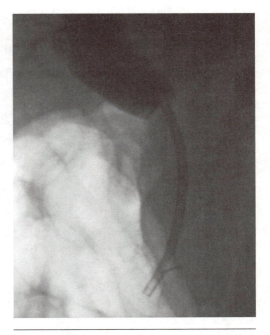

Figure 21.9. Endoscopic cholangiogram images of a patient with a pancreatic carcinoma. A stent has been successfully placed.

duct. The lower end of the common duct can be the most difficult area to visualize with transabdominal ultrasound but sometimes a pancreatic mass will be identified and, if choledocholithiasis is present, calculi will be visualized within the duct in about 70–80% of patients by an expert operator.

Regardless of the apparent level of obstruction on ultrasound, the next investigation is generally an endoscopic cholangiogram (ERC), particularly if it is believed that intervention (stone extraction or stent insertion) will be required (*Figure 21.9*). Noninvasive or less invasive techniques including MRCP, CT cholangiography (CTC) and EUS are increasingly available, and may have a role in planning subsequent intervention, but the therapeutic potential of ERCP gives it a clear advantage in the context of jaundice.

ERCP will be technically impossible or unsuccessful in a small proportion of patients and direct PTC remains a valuable technique in this situation (*Figure 21.10*). PTC also provides the option of proceeding to stent insertion in the case of malignant strictures. Percutaneous management of bile duct calculi is more difficult and only rarely appropriate, but the insertion of a temporary biliary drain can be life-saving in a patient with severe cholangitis and will allow time for planning subsequent surgery (*Figure 21.11*) or a further attempt at ERCP.

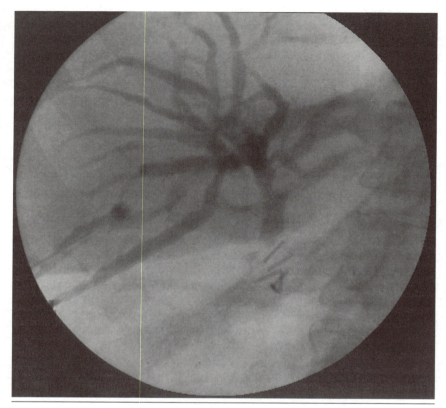

Figure 21.10. Percutaneous transhepatic cholangiography in a patient with bile duct obstruction due to clipping of the common bile duct at laparoscopic cholecystectomy.

When a malignant stricture has been demonstrated, the patient will be assessed as to the possibility of curative surgery. In this context, spiral CT is the principal technique employed at present, although MRI may take over this role as it becomes more widely available. If after optimal cross-sectional imaging the patient is thought suitable for curative resection, a laparoscopic ultrasound is often useful to exclude omental, mesenteric and liver lesions not detected on noninvasive imaging.

Dysphagia

Dysphagia should be distinguished from odynophagia, which is usually due to esophagitis. This is often secondary to gastroesophageal reflux but may also be due to infection, drugs, corrosives or CD. Upper GI endoscopy is the best test in these patients, allowing direct visualization of the mucosa and the detection of non-ulcerative inflammation as well as providing histological material from biopsy.

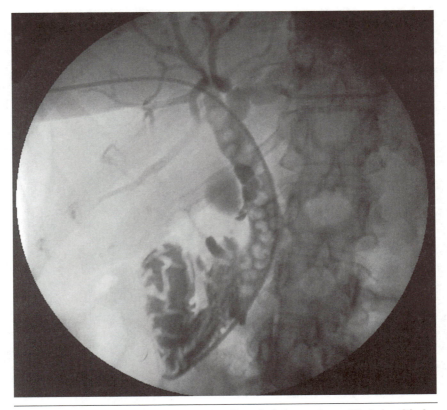

Figure 21.11. Percutaneous placement of a biliary drain in a patient with cholangitis due to multiple common duct stones.

Barium swallow remains the standard radiological investigation for patients with dysphagia. Patients are asked to swallow a barium suspension while rapid sequence or video images are taken of the pharynx in the frontal and lateral projections. Images of the rest of the esophagus are then obtained. This will show the site and length of any stricture (*Figure 21.12*). Patients with dysphagia who have a normal barium swallow should go on to have a marshmallow swallow. In this test, a 15-mm piece of marshmallow is swallowed with the liquid. This will stick at the level of a stricture, reproducing the patient's symptoms. Subtle strictures may only be identified by the use of this marshmallow swallow. If a stricture is demonstrated by the barium study, the patient should proceed to an upper GI endoscopy to allow a biopsy of the stricture to be obtained. In the past, the endoscopy had to wait for another day as the retained barium can block the scope channels. However, it has been shown that endoscopy can safely be performed on the same day if the patient is given 10 mg metoclopramide and a can of cola drink.

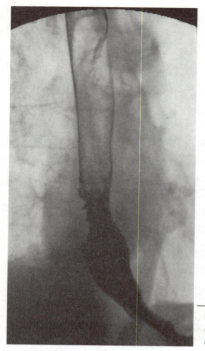

Figure 21.12. Barium swallow in a patient with dysphagia demonstrating an irregular distal esophageal stricture due to carcinoma.

If the dysphagia is due to an esophageal carcinoma, then further imaging is required to stage the tumor. A contrast-enhanced CT scan of the thorax and upper abdomen will help to show any local invasion and the presence of liver metastases or celiac nodes. CT is good at showing distal disease but local staging is unreliable. Local staging is best done by EUS. This will enable the tumor to be staged accurately and allow treatment to be optimized. Diagnostic EUS uses a radial ultrasound probe on the end of a side-viewing endoscope and allows visualization of the tumor and the layers of the esophageal wall.

If the tumor is considered amenable only to palliative treatment, then an expandable metal stent should be placed. These come in a variety of designs both covered and uncovered, and selection depends on the patient and the position of the tumor. As a growing number of these tumors are now at the gastroesophageal junction, some stents are now tapered in an attempt to reduce stent migration into the stomach. The stents can be placed under fluoroscopic (*Figure 21.13*) or endoscopic guidance, depending on local expertise and availability. After obtaining consent, the patient is sedated and a guide wire is placed across the stricturing tumor into the stomach under endoscopic or fluoroscopic control. Even tumors causing complete obstruction can be crossed in almost all cases using modern hydrophilic wires. The expandable stent is positioned over the wire and once in place is deployed. Patients can be discharged the following day unless there are complications and are often able to eat almost a normal diet.

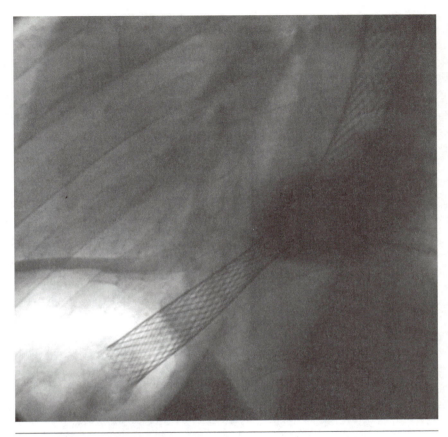

Figure 21.13. Images of a successfully placed esophageal stent.

Vomiting

Patients may present with vomiting due to metabolic disturbances or obstruction. The diagnosis of metabolic disturbances will depend on the history and biochemistry with little place for imaging. Imaging has a pivotal role in the diagnosis of vomiting due to obstruction. The imaging modalities used will depend on the patient's pre-existing condition and age. In the first 2 months of age, an ultrasound scan is the best test to make the diagnosis of hypertrophic pyloric stenosis. In adult patients, a plain erect CXR and supine abdominal film are the most appropriate first tests in most patients. The CXR may show mediastinal gas if the vomiting has resulted in an esophageal rupture (Boerhaave syndrome), while the abdominal film may show the site of any obstruction. Further examination will depend on the site and severity of the obstruction. In patients with gastric outlet obstruction, endoscopy can be very helpful but on occasion, a barium study may be required. Patients with gastric outlet obstruction due to an antral tumor will require CT staging but are often only suitable for palliative intervention. In the past this has been by means of a gastro-jejunostomy but increasingly, this is being replaced in frail patients by the placement of an expandable metallic stent across the tumor (*Figure 21.14*). This can be done solely using fluoroscopic control but a combination of endoscopy and fluoroscopy can make the placement easier. When successful the response to these stents is dramatic with the vomiting ceasing almost immediately and the patients returning to a normal diet on the following day.

In patients with small bowel obstruction, a CT scan is the best modality for further evaluation and can demonstrate the site and cause of the obstruction as well as demonstrating complications such as local perforation or ischemia. In patients with intermittent vomiting or subacute obstruction due to a small bowel abnormality, the best test is a small bowel enteroclysis. This test involves the placement of a tube through the nose into the jejunum. Barium is then pumped through the tube at carefully controlled rates to provide images of the small bowel. Enteroclysis delivers high flow rates of barium to the small bowel and can demonstrate the presence of subtle strictures by the observation of dilated bowel loops above and collapsed bowel loops below the lesion. The obstructing lesion itself can usually be characterized or adhesions diagnosed by a characteristic tethering of bowel loops at the site.

Diarrhea

Diarrhea may be due to infective causes and these should be excluded first partic-ularly when there are other relevant pointers in the history. Once this has been

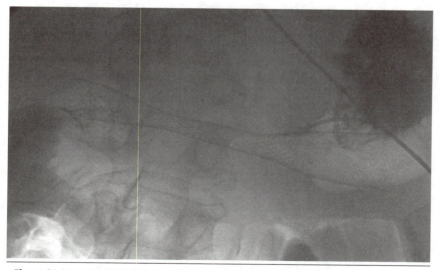

Figure 21.14. Image showing the successful placement of a gastroduodenal stent. This was placed because of gastric outflow obstruction caused by a carcinoma.

excluded, imaging depends on the most likely differential diagnosis. In patients in whom noninfective colitis is suspected, a colonoscopy allows biopsies to determine the histological diagnosis and assess the extent and severity of disease. When this is not possible, a combination of a flexible sigmoidoscopy and a barium enema can be used but this will tend to underestimate the extent of the colitis.

If CD is suspected, a small bowel meal with pneumocolon is the best test to evaluate the small bowel anatomy. In this test, the patient is given barium to drink and abdominal films are taken at intervals as the barium passes through the small bowel. Spot views with compression of the bowel are taken if there are any suspicious areas on the abdominal films. Once barium has reached the colon, further compression films are taken particularly of the terminal ileum and then gas is insufflated into the rectum. This should provide exquisite images of the terminal ileum (*Figure 21.15*). Other abnormalities of the small bowel causing diarrhea, such as jejunal diverticulosis or radiation ileitis, can also be demonstrated with

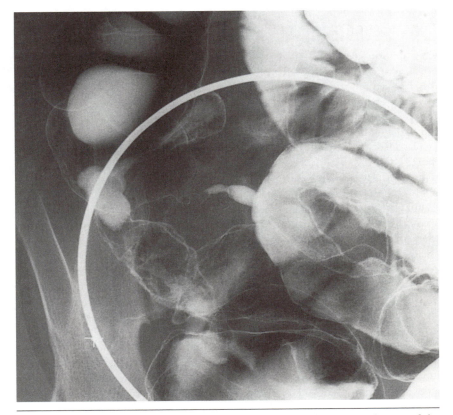

Figure 21.15. Small bowel meal with rectal gas to provide double contrast images of the terminal ileum. This is narrowed and ulcerated due to Crohn's disease.

this small bowel meal examination. More subtle changes, particularly to the jejunum, may require a small bowel enteroclysis for optimal demonstration.

In patients with diarrhea from gastrinoma, imaging is targeted at identifying the islet cell tumor. This is in the pancreas in almost 90% of cases and will usually appear as a high-attenuation mass on CT, following intravenous contrast. An arterial phase scan on a single or (preferably) multidetector CT scanner gives the best chance of detecting the lesion. MRI and EUS can also be useful in locating the tumor but if these fail, selective angiography should be requested.

In patients with diarrhea and flushing where carcinoid tumor is suspected, CT of the abdomen may show both the primary lesion and liver secondaries. If no liver abnormality is shown and suspicion remains high, then somatostatin receptor scintigraphy (an octreotide scan) can demonstrate metastases in the liver and elsewhere in the abdomen. PET scanning can also be extremely useful when available. In patients who are getting severe symptoms due to carcinoid deposits despite maximal therapy, the lesions can be treated by embolization or high-activity radiolabeled octreotide therapy.

Constipation

Constipation is a term that covers a multitude of clinical presentations. In the acute setting of a patient with vomiting and absolute constipation due to bowel obstruction, the plain abdominal film will usually show the level of the obstruction but seldom the cause. Dilatation of small bowel loops with a collapsed colon indicates small bowel or cecal obstruction and surgery to relieve the obstruction is usually required. A definitive preoperative diagnosis can often be obtained with an abdominal CT scan, which can demonstrate the presence of masses as well as hernias, bowel ischemia and closed-loop obstruction. In patients in whom there is some uncertainty about the need for urgent surgery, a plain abdominal film taken 4 h after 100 ml of oral gastrograffin can be very useful. This is particularly helpful if the patient has had prior surgery and adhesions are a possible diagnosis. If contrast has reached the colon on the 4-h film then conservative management is likely to be successful. If there is dilatation of small and large bowel in the acute setting, the diagnosis is likely to be between colonic obstruction or a metabolic disturbance leading to pseudo-obstruction. Careful evaluation of the images by a radiologist may help to differentiate between these but often an unprepared single contrast enema is required. This will show either an obstructing lesion or, in the case of pseudo-obstruction, free flow of contrast into the dilated portion of bowel.

Patients with a change in bowel habit characterized by increasing constipation may occasionally have a colonic carcinoma that is beginning to cause luminal narrowing. In these patients, the colon should be investigated with either a flexible sigmoidoscopy and barium enema or a colonoscopy.

The majority of patients with long-standing constipation will have transit disorders or pelvic floor dysfunction. Slow transit can be detected with a shape

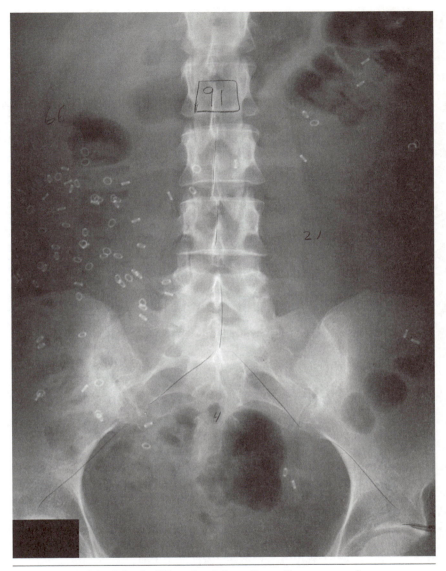

Figure 21.16. Plain abdominal film taken 5 days after radio-opaque markers were ingested. The large number remaining in the colon indicates slow transit.

study (*Figure 21.16*), in which patients take a capsule containing radio-opaque markers. A plain abdominal film at 5 days will show whether the transit is normal. In those patients with pelvic floor dysfunction, imaging investigations include defecating proctography (*Figure 21.17*), endoanal ultrasound and MRI.

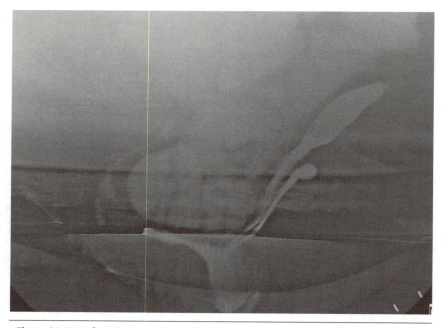

Figure 21.17. Defecating proctogram that demonstrates an enterocele, rectocele and rectal intussusception.

The patient with ascites

As in most other gastroenterological problems, the first imaging investigation will be an ultrasound scan. Ultrasound is extremely sensitive in the detection of even small volumes of ascites. The circulation of peritoneal fluid around the peritoneal cavity and the negative pressure created by diaphragmatic movement during respiration mean that when only a small volume of ascites is present it will generally be seen around the liver, regardless of cause. With increasing volumes of ascites, fluid will be seen to accumulate in the pelvis and in the flanks.

When the presence of ascites has been confirmed with ultrasound, the next step is to determine whether this is due to malignancy. Ascitic fluid is generally trans-sonic, in other words clear on ultrasound. If there are echoes within the fluid, this may suggest the presence of hemorrhage, infection or chylous ascites. Rarely, a malignant exudate may be sufficiently proteinaceous to cause the fluid to appear turbid.

Peritoneal and omental thickening and nodularity, which are the hallmarks of peritoneal malignancy, are generally very difficult to identify on ultrasound. Clearly there may be clinical factors or other pointers such as the presence of hepatic lesions, splenomegaly, portal or hepatic venous thrombosis, which may help to suggest the cause of the ascites.

Having confirmed the presence of ascites on ultrasound, if there is no readily apparent cause, the portal and hepatic venous systems should be assessed with Doppler. The patency of the portal vein and direction and rate of flow within, the presence of thrombus and the presence or absence of collateral vessels can all be assessed. Similarly, the hepatic veins should be scrutinized to exclude veno-occlusive disease.

If there is still no cause apparent, the next investigation should be a CT scan, which is very much more sensitive than ultrasound in determining the presence of peritoneal thickening and nodularity. Although there are rare benign causes of this such as tuberculous peritonitis, which should be considered in at-risk patients, the identification of peritoneal thickening on CT strongly suggests a malignant cause for the ascites. Ovarian cancer is the most likely primary in women. In men, gastric, pancreatic and colonic cancer can all present in this way.

Paracentesis will usually confirm the diagnosis in a patient with malignant ascites and can also be used to exclude peritonitis. If only a small volume of fluid is present, ultrasound or CT can be used for guidance.

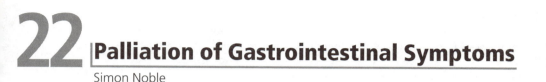

22 Palliation of Gastrointestinal Symptoms

Simon Noble

Introduction

Changing role of palliative care

Gastroenterology teams are seeing an increasing number of patients with malignancy and a successful service should involve managing common symptoms and appropriate referral to local palliative care teams. The old palliative care model (see *Figure 22.1*) excluded palliative care input until active curative treatment was no longer appropriate. At this point, care would be handed over to palliative care teams until death. This model makes the false assumption that common symptoms, such as nausea, anorexia, constipation, pain and so on, only occur in the terminal stages. The modern model (see *Figure 22.2*) attempts to dovetail palliative care with active treatment, gradually increasing its involvement as active treatment seems less appropriate. Some disease processes, for example carcinoma of the pancreas, are likely to require palliative care input early after diagnosis.

Figure 22.1. Traditional model of palliative care showing set point at which active treatment ceases and comfort-only begins.

Figure 22.2. Modern model of palliative care showing gradual introduction of increasing palliative care as active treatment becomes less appropriate.

Common misconceptions

Only a small proportion of patients with incurable cancer are looked after by palliative care teams and this may be due to an unwillingness of the acute team to refer. This unwillingness may come from a concern that palliative care teams will allow patients with reversible pathology to die, adopting a 'comfort-only' approach rather than active treatment where appropriate.

Making the most of the palliative care team

Palliative care teams are used to offering advice on symptoms and often this can be done over the phone. Some patients with symptoms that are difficult to control may need admitting to a specialist palliative care unit for a short while. This should not be considered a 'death sentence', as 50% of palliative care inpatients will be discharged home after an average length of stay of 13 days. Close liaison with the team will enable you to see for yourself what facilities and skills the team has to offer, in addition to remaining involved in your patient's care. It is commonly our practice to remain in close contact with the patient's referring team so that management decisions can be made in a consensual manner, having considered all options.

Palliative care teams pay attention to the psychosocial aspects of symptoms as well as the physical. It is idealistic to think we are able to address all a patient's psychological issues in a short follow-up clinic; however, it is worth knowing that over 50% of cancer outpatients are likely to have symptoms of depression if carefully looked for. Most will respond to simple antidepressants and psychological support. This chapter does not suggest we should devote busy, overcrowded clinics to counseling every patient we see, but we should at least have a high index of suspicion that our patients might well be depressed and may need referring back to their GP for assessment.

What this chapter is and is not

This chapter will not turn you into a fully-fledged palliative care physician. It hopes to give you some pointers as how best to approach common symptoms faced by patients with advanced GI malignancy and the drugs that may be considered in these situations. Palliative care physicians are used to prescribing drugs for unlicensed indications and at unusual doses. Therefore, it should be noted that drug treatments suggested here are often not in their recognized doses or uses.

Management approach to some common problems

Pain control

Pain should be carefully assessed with a full history and examination. Analgesics should be prescribed according to the mechanism of the pain. Bony pain may respond better to an NSAID, whilst neuropathic pain may need an anti-convulsant, for example sodium valproate. The World Health Organization's analgesic ladder should be considered when treating cancer-related pain:

- Nonopioid and/or adjuvants
- Weak opioid and/or adjuvants
- Strong opioid and/or adjuvants

For difficult pains, we recommend taking advice from the local palliative care team, but the following facts about morphine may help tease out some of the more common problems:

- When initially prescribing morphine, start a regular antiemetic and laxative at the same time
- Review response to the opioid regularly and increase the dose as required
- There is no ceiling to the dose of morphine that can be given and many patients on long-term morphine will have escalating requirements
- When increasing the dose, do so by increments of 30–50%
- Divide the total 24-h dose of morphine used by 2 and convert to a twice-daily dose of slow-release morphine, for example, MST
- For breakthrough pain, give one-sixth the total 24-h dose, for example for a patient on 120 mg b.d. of MST, the breakthrough dose of morphine will be 240 mg divided by 6 = 40 mg
- The equivalent subcutaneous dose of diamorphine is a third of the oral morphine dose, for example 150 mg oral morphine = 50 mg subcutaneous diamorphine

Constipation

Constipation is a common symptom facing cancer patients. Prevention is better than cure, since it can have many complications:

- Abdominal pain/colic
- Intestinal obstruction
- Urinary retention
- Overflow diarrhea

There are a number of common causes of constipation in patients with advanced GI malignancy:

- Drugs, for example opioids, tricyclics, antacids, phenothiazines and so on
- Dehydration
- Abdominal wall muscle paresis, for example from spinal cord compression
- Hypercalcemia
- Primary or secondary bowel disease

In a patient with cancer, these causes should be considered, and if appropriate, treated.

When treating a patient with constipation, general measures should be first introduced, such as increasing fluid intake, high-fiber diet and improved mobility. Various laxatives are available (*Box 22.1*) and should be chosen carefully depending on the need for bowel stimulation or stool softening. Typical starting doses are given but should be titrated up to achieve appropriate results.

Choice of laxatives varies in different units. It is often our practice to use a combination of senna/magnesium hydroxide, with a typical dose of 10 mg/10 ml b.d., although the choice of laxative should be tailored to an individual patient's needs.

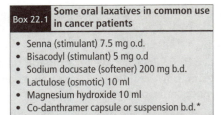

Box 22.1 **Some oral laxatives in common use in cancer patients**

- Senna (stimulant) 7.5 mg o.d.
- Bisacodyl (stimulant) 5 mg o.d
- Sodium docusate (softener) 200 mg b.d.
- Lactulose (osmotic) 10 ml
- Magnesium hydroxide 10 ml
- Co-danthramer capsule or suspension b.d.*

*Can cause a sore perianal rash and colors urine orange.

Colic

Painful spasm of smooth muscle may lead to intestinal colic. If possible, stop any drugs which may be causing these symptoms, such as stimulant laxatives or prokinetic antiemetics (e.g. metoclopramide). Then consider using Buscopan® 40–90 mg s.c. in 24 h or Mebeverine 135 mg t.d.s. orally. Buscopan is available as an oral preparation but is poorly absorbed and best avoided.

Diarrhea

The common causes of diarrhea in cancer patients are listed as follows:

- *Clostridium difficile*
- Acquired lactose intolerance
- Radiotherapy-induced
- Drugs, for example NSAIDs, laxatives

Box 22.2 **Drugs used for the symptomatic control of diarrhea**

- Codeine 30–60 mg p.o. q.d.s.
- Loperamide 2 mg (1 cap) p.o. q.d.s. The dose can be increased to 16 mg daily, although higher doses are occasionally used
- Octreotide 300 µg s.c. in 24 h. The dose can be increased to 1200 µg in 24 h

It is worth remembering that opioids are constipating and diarrhea may occur on decreasing the dose or converting to an alternative opioid such as fentanyl. For symptomatic control of diarrhea, consider the drugs in *Box 22.2.*

Nausea and vomiting

This is a common symptom in many malignancies, not just GI. It is beyond the scope of this chapter to cover all aspects of the management of nausea and vomiting in advanced malignancy, as the causes are often multifactorial and treatment complex, but the following principles should be kept in mind.

(1) Identify the specific causes of nausea and vomiting:
  - Constipation
  - Gastritis
  - Raised intracranial pressure
  - Oropharyngeal candida
  - Hypercalcemia
  - Drugs-induced, for example morphine

2   Choose an antiemetic based on the most likely cause of the nausea and vomiting:
    − Drugs or metabolic − haloperidol
    − Gastric stasis − metoclopramide
    − GI tract involvement − cyclizine
    − Cerebral tumor − cyclizine
3   If vomiting is preventing drug absorption, use an alternative route of administration, for example syringe driver
4   Check blood electrolytes and calcium
    − Uremia − consider fluids or lowering dose of opioids
    − Hypercalcemia − can be treated with intravenous fluids and bisphosphonates
5   If the first drug of choice has not worked, consider another antiemetic from a different group. If the first drug of choice was *partially* effective, consider *adding* another antiemetic from a different group.
    − Cyclizine 150 mg and haloperidol 2.5 mg in 24 h is often an effective combination
    − Methotrimeprazine (Levomepromazine) acts at several receptor sites and alone may replace previous unsuccessful combinations
    − Dexamethasone 4 mg daily often contributes an antiemetic effect of unknown mechanism
6   Always give antiemetics regularly.
7   Do not prescribe cyclizine with metoclopramide as cyclizine's antimuscarinic effects will inhibit the prokinetic action of metoclopramide.
8   The patient's clinical condition will change over time, and response to antiemetics should be regularly reviewed.

Hiccups

Several drugs have been used for hiccups but none are consistently reliable. If hepatic metastases are thought to be a factor, consider using dexamethasone, which is often effective. Where gastric distension is thought to be the cause, the following may be used:

- Asilone® 10 ml p.r.n.
- Metoclopramide 10 mg t.d.s.
- Nifedipine 5 mg t.d.s. p.r.n.

Other drugs that can be used for more persistent hiccups include:

- Baclofen 5 mg t.d.s.
- Chlorpromazine 25–50 mg nocte

To achieve an effect a sedative dose needs to be given, hence the nocturnal dosing.

Mouth pain

Mouth pain is common in patients with advanced malignancy. Causes to be considered and treatment options are listed in *Box 22.3*.

Box 22.3 Causes and treatment options for mouth pain	
Common causes of mouth pain	**Treatment options**

• Local tumor
• Bacterial infections
• Oral candida
• Herpes simplex
• Post radiotherapy / chemotherapy mucositis
	• Treat any specific cause.
	• For generalized pain
	  – Difflam®, Mucaine®, oral opioids
	• Localized pain
	  – Bonjela® oral gel, Adcortyl® in Orabase, lignocaine gel
	For post radiotherapy/chemotherapy mucositis we have had success with cocaine mouthwashes

Anorexia

Anorexia is a common part of the cancer-induced anorexia–cachexia syndrome. Forty per cent of patients are likely to respond to corticosteroids. When corticosteroids are contraindicated, progestagens may be as affective but more expensive. The drugs most commonly used are dexamethasone 8 mg orally or s.c. o.d. (lower doses can be used initially) and megestrol acetate 160 mg o.d.

Reversible causes of poor appetite should also be considered and treated if appropriate:

* Nausea
* Candidiasis
* Dysphagia
* Esophagitis/esophageal spasm

Other difficult problems

Fistulae

Fistulae are sometimes encountered in patients with large and small bowel tumors. Fistulae can cause significant problems with wound care and significantly impair the patient's quality of life. Octreotide helps reduce secretions in the small bowel and reduces intestinal motility. It is a useful treatment for patients with high-output fistulae and should be used in a dose of 300 µg s.c. in 24 h. This can be increased up to 1200 µg in 24 h if necessary.

Oral candida

Eighty per cent of patients with metastatic disease will have oral candida, but not necessarily be symptomatic. Candidiasis may present with:

- Dry mouth
- Altered taste
- Smooth reddened tongue
- Soreness
- Dysphagia
- Angular chelitis
- Furred tongue

Confirmation by routine swabs is rarely necessary. Regular oral hygiene is essential and dentures must be thoroughly cleaned. The treatment of candidiasis is given in *Box 22.4*:

Ascites

Within the palliative care setting, malignant ascites should be treated if it is causing discomfort, dyspnea or vomiting. Paracentesis is the most effective way of removing fluid but repeated procedures carry increased risk of complications. Some cancer patients may benefit from repeated paracentesis for months. Prognosis is poor when patients are requiring drainage less than every 14 days.

Diuretics do have a role in the management of malignant ascites and a combination of a loop diuretic with spironolactone will achieve the best results. Palliative care patients are sensitive to changes in blood biochemistry and we recommend regular monitoring of electrolytes to ensure the patient is not becoming hypokalemic or developing renal failure.

Intestinal obstruction

Intestinal obstruction is often precipitated in palliative care by constipation. Careful use of stimulant laxatives and rectal interventions may resolve the matter. The clinical features suggestive of obstruction in these patients include:

- Presence of colic
- History of bowel not being opened
- Vomiting relieves nausea
- Large volume vomitus

The definitive treatment for obstruction is surgery but this is often inappropriate in patients with advanced metastatic disease. Likewise, a large-bore nasogastric tube should be avoided if at all possible (and usually can be). Drug treatments for intestinal obstruction include:

- Cyclizine 150 mg + haloperidol 2.5 mg s.c. over 24 h to relieve nausea. Alternatively, consider methotrimeprazine 25 mg s.c. over 24 h if the patient needs mild anxiolytic or sedation

- Metoclopramide s.c. may be used to relieve partial bowel obstruction but may increase colic or vomiting in complete obstruction
- Insure adequate pain relief is given, using diamorphine as required
- Colic may be helped by buscopan® 20 mg s.c. stat followed by 40–80 mg s.c. over 24 h
- Dexamethasone 4 mg b.d. s.c. may help relieve the obstruction if due to high obstruction (gastric outlet) or lymphoma. However, addition of steroids will increase appetite which is not always welcomed in someone with obstruction.
- If vomiting remains frequent, consider adding octreotide 400–900 µg s.c. over 24 h to reduce the volume and frequency of vomitus.

Further reading

Twycross, R. (2001) *Symptom Management in Advanced Cancer.* 3rd edn. Radcliffe Medical Press, Abingdon.

Index